HEART DISEASE
IN PERSONS
WITH DOWN SYNDROME

HEART DISEASE
IN PERSONS
WITH DOWN SYNDROME

edited by

Bruno Marino, M.D.

and

Siegfried M. Pueschel, M.D., Ph.D., M.P.H.

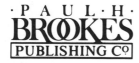 Baltimore • London • Toronto • Sydney

Paul H. Brookes Publishing Co.
Post Office Box 10624
Baltimore, Maryland 21285-0624

Typeset by PRO-IMAGE Corporation,
Techna-Type Division, York, Pennsylvania.
Manufactured in the United States of America by
The Maple Press Co., York, Pennsylvania.

Dr. Bruno Marino was supported by the Research N. 91/02/032 given by
Bambino Gesú Hospital and the National Council of Health of the Italian
government.

Library of Congress Cataloging-in-Publication Data
Heart disease in persons with Down syndrome / edited by Bruno Marino,
  Siegfried M. Pueschel.
      p.   cm.
    Includes selected papers from the International Congress on Heart
Disease in Down Syndrome, held in Rome, Italy, in May 1992, as well
as other invited contributions.
    Includes bibliographical references and index.
    ISBN 1-55766-224-X
    1. Congenital heart disease—Congresses.   2. Congenital heart
disease in children—Congresses.   3. Down's syndrome—
Complications—Congresses.   I. Marino, Bruno.   II. Pueschel,
Siegfried M.   III.   International Congress on Heart Disease in Down
Syndrome (1992: Rome, Italy)
      [DNLM: 1.   Heart Defects, Congenital—in adulthood.
2.   Down Syndrome—complications.   3.   Heart Diseases—
complications.   WG 220 H436   1995
RC687.H43   1996
616.1'2043—dc20
DNLM/DLC
for Library of Congress   95-24884
                                                                            CIP

British Library Cataloguing-in-Publication data are available from the British
Library.

CONTENTS

ABOUT THE EDITORS

Bruno Marino, M.D., is a pediatric cardiologist. He has worked at Bambino Gesú Hospital in Rome, Italy, since 1982. Dr. Marino graduated from the University La Sapienza of Rome, and specializes in cardiology and pediatrics. He perfected his training in pathology at the University of Padua, Italy; adult cardiology at the Catholic University of Rome; and pediatric cardiology at The Children's Hospital in Boston, Massachusetts.

Dr. Marino is a consultant in pediatric cardiology at Bambino Gesù Hospital and since 1982 he has been professor of congenital heart disease at the postgraduate school of cardiology at Catholic University of Rome, Italy. He has written several papers on anatomy and echocardiography, surgical treatment, and genetics of congenital heart diseases.

Siegfried M. Pueschel, M.D., Ph.D., M.P.H., as Director of The Child Development Center of Rhode Island Hospital since 1975, has worked with thousands of children with special needs. He has published 15 books about various developmental disabilities and has written more than 200 articles relating to many types of disabling conditions. Prior to his appointment at the Rhode Island Hospital, he initiated a lead poisoning program, became director of the first Down Syndrome Program, and provided leadership to the PKU and Inborn Errors of Metabolism Program at The Children's Hospital in Boston, Massachusetts.

Certified by the American Board of Pediatrics and a Diplomate of the American Board of Medical Genetics, his academic appointments include Lecturer in Pediatrics, Harvard Medical School; and Professor of Pediatrics, Brown University. During the past 25 years, Dr. Pueschel has been involved in clinical activities, research, and teaching; and he continues to pursue his interest in developmental disabilities, biochemical genetics, and chromosome abnormalities, particularly Down syndrome.

CONTRIBUTORS

Maitre Azcarate, M.J., M.D.
Jefe de Seccion
Servicio de Cardiologia Pediatrica
Hospital Ramon Y Cajal
Madrid 28034
SPAIN

Carol Bacchus, Dr.sc.hum.
Institute of Humangenetics and
  Anthropology
University of Heidelberg
Im Neuenheimer Feld 328
Heidelberg 69120
GERMANY

Yaron I. Bar-El, M.D.
Harvard Medical School
Children's Hospital
300 Longwood Avenue
Boston, Massachusetts 02115

John Burn, M.D., FRCP
Professor of Clinical Genetics
Department of Human Genetics
University of Newcastle upon Tyne
19/20 Claremont Palce
Newcastle upon Tyne NE2 4AA
GREAT BRITAIN

Werner Buselmaier, Dr.rer.nat
Institute of Humangenetics and
  Anthropology
University of Heidelberg
Im Neuenheimer Feld 328
Heidelberg 69120
GERMANY

Edward B. Clark, M.D.
Chief of Pediatric Cardiology
University of Rochester
School of Medicine and Dentistry
Box 631
601 Elmwood Avenue
Rochester, New York 14642

Duccio C. Di Carlo, M.D.
Associate in Cardiac Surgery
Pediatric Cardiac Surgery
Bambino Gesú Hospital
Piazza Sant'Onofrio 4
Rome 00165
ITALY

Robert M. Freedom, M.D.,
FRCPC
Professor of Pediatrics and
Pathology
The University of Toronto
Faculty of Medicine
The Hospital for Sick Children
Chief, Division of Cardiology
555 University Avenue
Toronto, Ontario M5G 1X8
CANADA

Carla Frescura, M.D.
Associate in Pathology
Department of Pathology
University of Padua
Via A. Gabelli 61
Padova 35121
ITALY

Judith A. Goodship, M.D., MRCP
Department of Human Genetics
University of Newcastle upon Tyne
19/20 Claremont Palce
Newcastle upon Tyne NE2 4AA
GREAT BRITAIN

Annemarie J.Y. Hofland, M.D.
Pediatric Oncology
Academic Medical Center
Meibergdreef 9
Amsterdam 1105 AZ
THE NETHERLANDS

Julie R. Korenberg, M.D.
Associate Professor of Pediatrics
UCLA, School of Medicine
Vice-Chair for Research, Pediatrics
Brawerman Chair of Molecular
  Genetics
Cedars-Sinai, Medical Center
Los Angeles, California 90048-0750

David N. Kurnit, M.D., Ph.D.
Professor of Pediatrics and Human
  Genetics
University of Michigan
Howard Hughes Medical Institute
Room 3520 MSRBI
1150 West Medical Center Drive
Ann Arbor, Michigan 48109

Hillel Laks, M.D.
Professor of Cardiothoracic Surgery
Chief, Cardiothoracic Surgery
UCLA, School of Medicine
10833 Le Conte Avenue
Los Angeles, California 90024-1741

Quero Jimenez Manuel, M.D.
Professor of Pediatrics
Chief, Pediatric Cardiology
Hospital Ramon Y Cajal
Madrid 28034
SPAIN

Consuelo Manrique Montilla, M.D.
Médicio Residente
Servicio de Cardiologia Pediatrica
Hospital Ramon Y Cajal
Madrid 28034
SPAIN

John Papagiannis, M.D.
Harvard Medical School
Children's Hospital
300 Longwood Avenue
Boston, Massachusetts 02115

Jeffrey M. Pearl, M.D.
Chief Resident
Cardiothoracic Surgery
UCLA, School of Medicine
10833 Le Conte Avenue
Los Angeles, California 90024-1741

Oscar A. Schwint, M.D.
Harvard Medical School
Children's Hospital
300 Longwood Avenue
Boston, Massachusetts 02115

James B. Seward, M.D.
Professor of Medicine and
    Pediatrics
Consultant in Cardiovascular
    Disease
Mayo Clinic
Rochester, Minnesota 55905

Gaetano Thiene, M.D., FRSC
Professor of Cardiovascular
    Pathology
Department of Pathology
University of Padua
Via A. Gabelli 61
Padova 35121
ITALY

Richard Van Praagh, M.D.
Director Cardiac Registry
Research Associate in Cardiology
Research Associate in Cardiac
    Surgery
Professor of Pathology
Harvard Medical School
Children's Hospital
300 Longwood Avenue
Boston, Massachusetts 02115

Flavia Ventriglia, M.D., Ph.D.
Research Fellow
Department of Pathology
University of Padua
Via A. Gabelli 61
Padova 35121
ITALY

Arnold C.G. Wenink, M.D.
Rijks Universiteit Leiden
Faculty of Medicine
Department of Anatomy
Wassenaarseweg 62 P.O. Box 9602
Leiden 2300 RC
THE NETHERLANDS

Lynne Wilson, B.Sc.
Department of Human Genetics
University of Newcastle upon Tyne
19/20 Claremont Palce
Newcastle upon Tyne NE2 4AA
GREAT BRITAIN

PREFACE

The diagnosis and treatment of congenital heart disease is of primary importance in the general health care of persons with Down syndrome. The high prevalence and the observed severity of congenital heart defects in many children with this chromosome disorder mandate an aggressive approach to diagnosis as well as to medical and surgical interventions available during early infancy; such an approach is necessary in order to prevent congestive heart failure, pulmonary vascular disease, and failure to thrive. Children with Down syndrome often have specific anatomic and physiologic cardiac problems and therefore require prompt attention.

Recent advances in basic cardiovascular research, diagnostic accuracy, and novel surgical approaches to persons with congenital heart disease have resulted in reduced mortality and morbidity in infants with Down syndrome. In this volume, these advances are discussed by foremost authorities in their respective fields of expertise. This book also documents the rapid changes in the knowledge base relating to genetic, investigative, and therapeutic aspects of congenital heart disease in Down syndrome.

In May 1992, an International Congress on Heart Disease in Down Syndrome was held in Rome, Italy. Participants at this meeting discussed the genetic, embryologic, anatomic, and physiologic aspects of congenital heart malformations in Down syndrome. In addition, diagnostic considerations, medical and surgical therapeutic management, and postoperative care and long-term follow-up were discussed. This volume is, however, not only a collection of the proceedings of this symposium; to present a well-rounded comprehensive view of heart disease in Down syndrome, this volume also includes other important papers by invited widely known investigators.

The goal of this book is to provide a state-of-the-art contribution to the field of congenital heart disease in Down syndrome. It will be particularly useful for pediatric cardiologists and pediatricians. Also, adult cardiologists, general practitioners, and various professionals working with children with Down syndrome will benefit from the knowledge imparted in this volume. Ultimately, the survival and the quality of life will be significantly enhanced if appropriate medical and surgical care is provided to all children with Down syndrome and congenital heart disease.

*To the memory
of my father,
Professor Mario Marino*

HEART DISEASE
IN PERSONS
WITH DOWN SYNDROME

HISTORICAL PERSPECTIVE OF HEART DISEASE IN PERSONS WITH DOWN SYNDROME

Siegfried M. Pueschel

ALTHOUGH JOHN LANGDON DOWN HAS been credited with first describing the condition that today bears his name (1), there were others, such as Esquirol in 1838 and Seguin in 1846, who prior to Down had pointed out certain characteristics in children with mental retardation that resembled those observed in persons with Down syndrome (2,3). Also, Duncan reported in 1866 a girl "with a small round head, Chinese-looking eyes, projecting a large tongue, who only knew a few words" (4). In the same year Down published a paper with the title *Observations on an Ethnic Classification of Idiots* (1). Apparently Down was so impressed by the similarity of children with this disorder that he felt a great need to describe these individuals in more detail. In his paper Down stated:

The hair is not black, as in the real Mongol, but of a brownish colour, straight and scanty. The face is flat and broad, and destitute of prominence. The cheeks are roundish, and extended laterally. The eyes are obliquely placed, and the internal canthi more than normally distant from one another. The palpebral fissure is very narrow. The forehead is wrinkled transversely from the constant assistance which the levatores palpebrarum derive from the occipitofrontalis muscle in the opening of the eyes. The lips are large and thick with transverse fissures. The tongue is long, thick, and is much roughened. The nose is small. The skin has a slight dirty yellowing tinge, and is deficient in elasticity, giving the appearance of being too large for the body (p. 3) (1).

In his further description, Down focused on behavioral issues as well as on the social and language development of such children. The only reference Down made to the cardiovascular system is his observation that "the circulation is feeble" (1).

As mentioned above, children with the syndrome had been recognized by other investigators prior to his report; however, Down deserves credit for describing some of the classic features of the children, thus distinguishing them from others with mental retardation, in particular those with cretinism. Down's great contribution was his recognition of specific physical characteristics and his description of the condition as a distinct and separate entity (1).

Down went beyond the mere description of the features of these children when he stated that "the boy's aspect is such that it is difficult to realize that he is the child of Europeans, but so frequently are these characters presented, that there can be no doubt that these ethnic features are the result of degeneration." According to Down the "mongoloid" features in the Caucasian child with this disorder were proof to him that "these examples of the result of degeneracy among mankind appear to me to furnish some arguments in favour of the unity of the human species" (1).

During the same year that Down's paper (1) appeared in the literature, Seguin published his book *Idiocy and Its Treatment by the Physiological Method* (5). Although Seguin had previously recognized children with this syndrome (3), he mentioned them again in his 1866 publication (5). In contrast to Down, Seguin did not think that these children had any resemblance to people of the Mongolian race. He called the condition "furfuraceous cretinism" (5). He stated that these children have "milk-white, rosy and peeling skin, with its shortcomings of all the integuments which give an unfinished aspect of the truncated fingers and nose; with its cracked lips and tongue; with its red ectopic conjunctiva, coming out to supply the curtailed skin at the margin of the lids" (5). Shuttleworth also disagreed with Down's observation of the mongoloid features of persons with this disorder (6). He pointed out the "striking divergencies between the physical characteristic of the real Mongol or Kalmuc and these mongoloid specimens of the Caucasian race" (6).

In 1876, Fraser and Mitchell, who had not been aware of Down's report, published a paper providing scientific data on 62 individuals with Down syndrome (7). In another publication, Mitchell emphasized their short life span, the observed brachycephaly, and that "their mental state is as distinct as peculiar" (8). He continued: "If the patients were brought together they would be found to resemble each other strikingly in personal appearance" (8). In both publications the cardiovascular aspects of persons with Down syndrome were not mentioned (7,8). Likewise Ireland in his book *Idiocy and Imbecility* did not refer to the cardiovascular system in individuals with Down syndrome (9).

In 1886 Shuttleworth classified mental retardation as congenital and noncongenital (i.e., developmental, accidental or acquired, and mixed causes) (6). He indicated that

> there is a remarkable variety of imbecility, probably scrofulous in its essence, which has obtained from its physiognomical characters the name of the "Mongol" or "Kalmuc" type. We have numerous specimens of that type in this institution (perhaps 3 per cent of its population); and you will notice in all a certain family resemblance, though they come from widely distant parts of our district. They all have a skin coarse in epidermis, if not furfuraceous; many have sore eye-lids, some fissured lips; but one of their most striking peculiarities is the state of the tongue, which is transversely fissured and has hypertrophied papillæ. Many of them have almond-shaped eyes obliquely set; and this feature, with the squat nose and wiry hair, give the "Mongol" aspect whence they derive their name. My view is that they are, in fact, unfinished children, and that their peculiar appearance is really that of a phase of fœtal life. I do not mean that they are necessarily prematurely born, but some cause has depressed the maternal powers, and there has been a defect of formative force. It is remarkable that, in our experience, nearly half these children are the last born of a long family; and in more than one-third a phthisical history has been traced. They are generally delicate in body, and very susceptible to cold; mentally, they have good imitative powers, are often very fond of music, and dance and drill well. Comparatively few grow up to be men and women; and, as a rule, they die of phthisis before 20 (p. 185) (6).

Again, in Shuttleworth's paper no mention is made of congenital heart disease in children with Down syndrome (6).

In the last decade of the nineteenth century, Garrod published several papers in which for the first time congenital heart disease was documented to be associated with Down syndrome (10–13). In his paper *On the Association of Cardiac Malformations with Other Congenital Defects,* Garrod described a patient named Annie M. who

> had been blue from birth, and when seen was very cyanotic, and had conspicuous clubbing of the fingers and toes; the nose was also blue and clubbed. A systolic murmur was heard all over the cardiac area in front, and also over the back of the chest. The child showed evident signs of mental deficiency, could not stand, and was spiteful and strange at times. Her countenance was that characteristic of the "Mongol" type of idiocy. She was subject to fits, which occurred about every alternate day, in the

course of which her colour became very dark, and her tongue, which was protruded from her mouth, was almost black (p. 54) (10).

As a scientist, Garrod was interested in the etiology of the congenital heart disease and discussed the then-prevalent theories including rheumatic fever and fetal endocarditis as causative factors.

In a meeting of the Clinical Society of London, Garrod presented "a child who displayed the typical Mongol caste features in association with a considerable degree of cyanosis and a loud systolic murmur best heard to the left of the sternum, about the middle of the cardiac area. She had been under observation for 8 months. At the seat of maximum murmur there was a perceptible thrill" (11). In a later meeting of the Clinical Society of London, Garrod presented another "five cases in which congenital cardiac lesions were met with in idiots of the Mongolian type" (12). During the same meeting other physicians also reported on children with Down syndrome and congenital heart disease.

In a subsequent publication Garrod dwelt further on the association of congenital heart disease with the "Mongolian form of idiocy" (13). He mentioned that

> cases which have come under my observation during the past few years have led me to believe that a special connection exists between congenital heart disease and that form of imbecility which is characterized by the "Mongolian" type of countenance. It is in no way surprising that two such congenital defects should be met within the same subject, for in a considerable proportion of cases of congenital heart disease associated malformations are present, either of external parts or of the internal viscera (p. 6) (13).

In addition to Annie M., whom he had described previously, Garrod reported the histories of four other children with Down syndrome who also had congenital heart disease. Garrod pointed out the phenotypic characteristics of these children and described the cardiovascular findings in more detail. In Stanley C. he observed

> a well-marked cyanosis of the skin and mucous membranes, which becomes greatly intensified when the child cries. The fingers and toes are not obviously clubbed. Their heart's apex-beat lies about an inch outside the nipple line. The cardiac dulness cannot be traced to the right of the sternum. A systolic thrill is palpable all over the precordial area, and a loud systolic murmur is heard which has its maximum intensity to the left of the sternum, at about the fourth interspace. The murmur is certainly less loud in the aortic and pulmonic areas (p. 6–7) (13).

In another child, R.R., Garrod noted that

> the limits of the cardiac dulness are not easily made out. There is a blowing systolic murmur heard all over the cardiac area, having its maximum

intensity in the pulmonic area, where also the second sound is markedly accentuated. At the aortic base the second sound is feeble (p. 7) (13).

In Lily J., Garrod observed

well-marked cyanosis, and the fingers and toes are clubbed. The heart's apex-beat lies just outside the nipple line, and the cardiac dulness extends about an inch to the right of the sternum. No thrill is felt, but a loud systolic murmur is heard over a wide area having its maximum intensity at the pulmonic base, but is also heard loudly below the right clavicle. The second sound is accentuated in the pulmonic area (p. 7) (13).

The last patient described in this paper is Annie P., who was noted

to be blue at times. . . . The heart's apex lies half an inch outside the nipple line; the dulness cannot be traced to the right of the sternum. At the apex a harsh, whiffing systolic murmur is heard, but there is no thrill, and the murmur is not conducted towards the base of the heart (p. 6) (13).

Garrod went on to discuss the prevalence of congenital heart disease in persons with Down syndrome (13). He mentioned that "one might reasonably expect that the far wider field of a large idiot asylum would afford numerous examples of the association in question. This is, however, not the case" (13). Apparently Garrod had contact with numerous physicians in charge of institutions, then called idiot asylums, and these physicians did not report an increased prevalence of congenital heart disease in their patients. Garrod speculated that most children with Down syndrome and with severe congenital heart disease had died during infancy or early childhood and that the ones seen in residential facilities were those who survived and who did not have cardiac defects (13).

In the same paper, Garrod continued to report on other patients with Down syndrome and congenital heart disease made known to him by his colleagues (13). He mentioned a patient brought to his attention by Smith who had found that "the heart is undersized and weak in these patients." Garrod also commented about his discussions with Thompson who "has very kindly supplied me with further information about . . . three patients. All of them were under four years of age, all were girls. . . . A postmortem examination in one case showed extreme tricuspid incompetence." Apparently Thompson had seen 13 children with Down syndrome, three of whom had congenital heart disease (13).

Although Garrod's scientific pursuits were primarily in the area of inborn errors of metabolism (a term that he coined), he surely had a keen interest in cardiovascular functions in youngsters with mental retardation and thus initiated the study of congenital heart disease in persons with Down syndrome.

Another early pioneer was Shuttleworth, who not only was involved in public policy issues relating to "the care and control of the feeble-minded" but also provided detailed phenotypic descriptions of persons with Down syndrome (14). Shuttleworth mentioned that "the heart is found incompletely finished not infrequently in children of this type, the foramen ovale remaining patent, and defects existing also in the intraventricular septum" (14). In 1903, Muir analyzed 26 cases of Down syndrome, and a year later Fennel presented three children with Down syndrome who had various malformations of the heart (15,16).

In the first few decades of this century several monographs on Down syndrome were published that also discussed cardiac findings in children with this chromosome disorder. Siegert and later Van der Scheer as well as Brousseau and Brainerd published works on Down syndrome that summarized information available on the subject at that time (17–19). There were other physicians in the early part of the twentieth century who contributed to the literature on Down syndrome, such as Bourneville, Comby, and Babonneix in France who made observations on many individuals with Down syndrome (20–22). Alberti in Italy, Hjorth in Denmark, and Neumann and Siegert in Germany also made substantial contributions expanding the knowledge about Down syndrome (17,23–25). Although these and other authors mainly focused on the epidemiology, etiology, and phenotypic descriptions of Down syndrome, they also discussed cardiac findings in individuals with this chromosome disorder. Despite the many descriptions of both clinical and postmortem findings of the heart in children with Down syndrome, it was not until 1924 that Abbott first reported the most commonly observed congenital heart malformation in Down syndrome, namely, the atrioventricular canal (26).

To summarize, since Garrod first investigated and described congenital heart disease in persons with Down syndrome, many other investigators in this field have provided additional information and more detailed descriptions of the association of congenital heart disease and Down syndrome. Hundreds of publications have focused on structural, pathogenetic, investigative, functional, and therapeutic aspects of congenital heart disease in children with Down syndrome. In particular, during the late 1900s, cardiac catheterization, new imaging techniques such as echocardiography, and novel cardiac surgical techniques ushered in the modern era of pediatric cardiology. We have experienced an explosion of knowledge in this field that is detailed in the chapters that follow.

REFERENCES

1. Down JLH. Observations on an ethnic classification of idiots. *London Hosp Clin Lect Rep.* 1866;3:259–262.
2. Esquirol JED. *Des maladies mentales considerees sous les rapports medical, hygienique et medico-legal.* [*Mental illness considered by the medical, health, and medical-legal reports*] Paris: Bailliére; 1838.
3. Seguin E. *Le traitement moral, l'hygiéne et l'éducation des idiots.* [*The moral treatment, hygiene and education of idiots*] Paris: Bailliére, 1846.
4. Duncan PM. *A Manual for the Classification, Training and Education of the Feeble-minded, Imbecile and Idiotic.* London: Longmans, Green & Co; 1866.
5. Seguin E. *Idiocy and Its Treatment by the Physiological Method.* New York: Wood; 1866.
6. Shuttleworth GE. Clinical lecture on idiocy and imbecility. *Br Med J* 1886;1:183–186.
7. Fraser J, Mitchell A. Kalmuc idiocy: report of a case with autopsy with notes on 62 cases by A. Mitchell. *J Ment Sci.* 1876;22:169–174.
8. Mitchell A. Notes on Kalmuc idiocy. *J Ment Sci.* 1876;22:174–179.
9. Ireland WW. *Idiocy and Imbecility.* London: Churchill; 1876.
10. Garrod AE. On the association of cardiac malformations with other congenital defects. *St. Bart Hosp Rep.* 1894;30:53–61.
11. Garrod AE. Cases illustrating the association of congenital heart disease with Mongolian form of idiocy. *Br Med J.* 1898;1:1255–1256.
12. Garrod AE. Congenital heart disease and the mongol type of idiocy. *Br Med J.* 1898;1:1200–1201.
13. Garrod AE. Association of congenital heart disease with the mongoloid form of idiocy. *Trans Clin Soc (London).* 1899;32:6–10.
14. Shuttleworth GE. Mongolian imbecility. *Br Med J.* 1909;1:661–663.
15. Muir J. An analysis of twenty-six cases of mongolism. *Arch Pediatr.* 1903;20:161–166.
16. Fennel CH. Mongolian imbecility. *J Ment Sci.* 1904;50:32–37.
17. Siegert F. Der Mongolismus. *Ergeb Inn Med Kinderh.* 1910;6:565–600.
18. Van der Scheer WM. Beiträge zur Kenntnis der mongoloiden Missbildung. *Abh Neuro Psychiat Psychol Grenzgeb.* 1927;41:1–8.
19. Brousseau K, Brainerd HG. *Mongolism: A Study of the Physical and Mental Characteristics of Mongolian Imbeciles.* London: Bailliére, Tindall & Cox; 1928.
20. Bourneville DM. L'idiotie du type mongolien. *Rech Clin Thérapeut Epilep.* 1902;22:136–142.
21. Comby J. Le mongolisme. *Arch Méd Enfant.* 1903;6:746–749.
22. Babonneix L. Contribution á l'étude anatomique de l'idiotie mongoliene. *Arch Méd Enfant.* 1909;12:497–501.
23. Alberti A. Un caso di idiozia mongoloide. *Giorn Psichiat Clin Tech.* 1904;32:335–339.
24. Hjorth B. On the etiology of mongolism. *J Ment Sci.* 1907;53:182–189.
25. Neumann H. Über den mongoloiden typus der idiotie. *Berl Klin Wochensch.* 1899;30:210–216.
26. Abbott ME. New accessions in cardiac anomalies. I. Pulmonary atresia of inflammatory origin. II. Persistent ostium primum with Mongolian idiocy. *Bull Int Assoc Med Mus.* 1924;10:111–117.

CHAPTER 2

GENETIC BASIS OF CONGENITAL HEART DISEASE IN DOWN SYNDROME

John Burn, Lynne Wilson, and Judith Goodship

NEARLY 500 YEARS HAVE ELAPSED since Leonardo da Vinci described an atrial septal defect (1). Progress in all aspects of pediatric cardiology has been dramatic, yet our understanding of causes that lead to cardiac malformations remains rudimentary. However, as the technology of molecular genetics advances, investigations become feasible. We have heard much about "reverse genetics" whereby genes are mapped or positioned on chromosomes, then sequenced and their functional role elucidated (2). In the case of congenital heart disease in Down syndrome we have an example of reverse reverse genetics because the first step toward cloning the gene responsible for atrioventricular septal defect (atrioventricular canal) was the recognition that trisomy 21 caused Down syndrome and that this otherwise rare malformation was strongly associated with the presence of an additional chromosome 21. We may deduce that duplication of one or more genes on chromosome 21 causes failure of the atrioventricular septum to form properly. Before examining this at the molecular genetic level, it is worthwhile to review the genetics of Down syndrome.

GENETICS OF DOWN SYNDROME

Down syndrome affects 1.3 per 1,000 live births (3). The incidence of live birth of infants with Down syndrome rises with maternal age such that a 40-year-old woman has about a 1% chance of having a child with Down syndrome. Nondisjunction in the first meiotic division of the oocyte is primarily responsible for the trisomic state (4). Failure at the second meiotic division in the female or at either step in the reduction division of male germ cells is less common. Molecular studies have reversed the suggestion, based on cytogenetic markers, that a significant proportion of infants with trisomy 21 were affected by paternal nondisjunction (5).

About 5% of patients with Down syndrome are associated with Robertsonian translocation, whereby one chromosome 21 becomes attached to another acrocentric chromosome, usually chromosome 14. It is thought that the chromosomes have sequences in common near the centromere, which leads to aberrant pairing. A mother who carries such a translocation has a 10% risk of giving birth to a child with trisomy 21 because the eggs are likely contain the free chromosome 21 and the other chromosome 21 is attached to chromosome 14. Trisomy 21 may also result from mosaicism in one of the parents, so that the cells responsible for gamete formation have three 21 chromosomes. Males with full trisomy 21 are probably always infertile (6). Women with Down syndrome may have children with a recurrence rate of about 1 in 3.

With the exception of the human Y chromosome and the mitochondrial chromosome, chromosome 21 is the smallest human chromosome. Along with chromosomes 13 and 18, chromosome 21 displays a relative excess of the bases adenine and thymine compared to guanine and cytosine. The relative lack of guanine and cytosine on these chromosomes suggests that relatively few genes are to be found on these chromosomes. This is likely to be one of the factors in their frequent survival to term. Trisomy may occur with any chromosome with the majority leading to very early pregnancy loss. The majority of cases of trisomy 21 are also spontaneously aborted early, so that the proportion reaching term bears little relationship to the true incidence of trisomy 21.

In several countries, screening for Down syndrome based on maternal serum levels of alphafetoprotein (AFP), human gonadotrophin (LCG), and oestriol is widely available (7–9). The test remains imprecise, with 5% of women being offered amniocentesis to detect two thirds of Down syndrome pregnancies. Inclusion of other markers such as urea resistant alkaline phosphatase (10) may improve detection in the future. Prenatal detection may also be based on recognition of nuchal thickening or heart malformation on ultrasound scan. Previously, 5% of children with heart defects had trisomy 21. This percentage will fall dramatically in countries where screening is used.

LOCALIZATION OF THE ATRIOVENTRICULAR SEPTAL DEFECT GENE ON CHROMOSOME 21

Korenberg et al. (11–13) made major progress in increasing our understanding of the cardiac genes on chromosome 21. These researchers investigated children with partial duplications and concluded that the gene or genes responsible for cardiac defects in Down syndrome are located near the tip of the long arm of chromosome 21. Korenberg et al. concluded that the candidate segment liable to produce heart malformation begins in q22.1 near marker D21S55 and extends to the tip or telomere (14,15). This is probably about 9 million bases (9 megabases, Mb). The key area may be further narrowed by comparison to the trisomy 16 murine map.

The mouse and human genomes display close similarities (16,17). There are genes on human chromosome 21 that correspond to genes on chromosome 16 in the mouse. Mouse heart embryos have features reminiscent of Down syndrome, and these mouse embryos have heart defects that frequently involve atrioventricular septal defect (18,19). Korenberg et al. (11–13) correlated the human and mouse maps and suggested that the area of greatest interest is the more proximal segment, which extends from D21S55 to Mx1, the influenza virus resistance gene (see Chapter 3). This may narrow the area to 5 Mb. In theory, such a segment could contain up to 5,000 genes but given their usual wide separation and the observation that this may be a relatively gene-poor chromosome, it may be assumed that the true number of genes is only a fraction of this total. Korenberg et al. suggested that as few as 30 genes may be present in the candidate segment.

MOLECULAR GENETIC STRATEGIES

With the evolution of the Human Genome Project, characterization of genes is occurring with increasing rapidity. Yeast artificial chromosome (YAC) libraries, chromosome microdissection, complementary DNA (cDNA) libraries with subtraction to determine tissue specificity, and multiple color fluorescent in situ hybridization to chromosomes are just a few of the techniques being used to identify and order genes. One difficulty, as more and more genes are identified, lies in the challenge of determining whether a particular gene is responsible for a particular malformation.

In the case of single-gene defects, such as cystic fibrosis or Duchenne muscular dystrophy, mutations in the coding segment of the candidate gene, particularly those that damage or prevent production of the gene product, provide evidence that the cystic fibrosis transmembrane conductance regulator and dystrophin genes, respectively, are the basis of the disease phenotypes. In the case of heart disease in Down syndrome it will be more difficult to decide which gene is responsible or whether a combination of gene defects is responsible for the cardiac defect. It is reasonable to assume that the gene will be expressed in the heart during the first trimester though expression may be transitory. Figure 1 shows an analysis of RNA, the product of gene transcription, in embryonic human hearts retrieved from therapeutic terminations. A radiolabeled probe for the collagen VI gene on chromosome 21 has produced a band on an autoradiograph at all gestations, which is in keeping with this gene being a candidate (20). The fact that it is a structural gene adds support. A major argument against this gene is that it does not map to chromosome 16 in the mouse, the segment homologous to human chromosome 21 (21), even though trisomy 16 mice develop AVSDs.

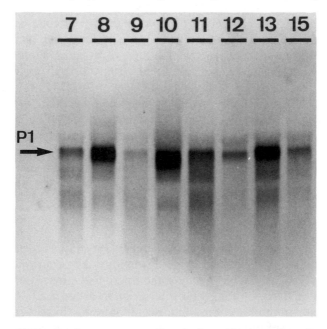

Figure 1. RNA studies demonstrate expression of collagen VI in human heart tissue from 7 to 15 weeks' gestation (13).

With the development of polymerase chain reaction, which permits amplification of very small quantities of DNA to levels that allow laboratory analysis, it will be possible to obtain complementary DNA probes from expressed genes in the endocardial cushions. The growth and/or adhesion of these cushions or the cellular structures in their immediate vicinity is highly likely to be implicated in the pathogenetic processes. Identification of genes expressed in the cushion region that are chromosome 21–specific should greatly reduce the number of genes of interest.

Elaborate analysis of heart cDNA libraries may be necessary because the relevant gene may be more widely expressed. Kurnit et al. (22) put forward the hypothesis that there was a failure to form the atrioventricular septum because the overexpression of a gene involved in cell adhesion led to premature cessation of growth (see Chapter 3). Some preliminary evidence was offered suggesting that this phenomenon could be reproduced in vitro in fibroblast culture. Were this to be confirmed it could be deduced that the gene responsible could be identified from a fibroblast cDNA library.

An alternative approach to the identification of candidate genes is to focus attention on families and individuals with apparently isolated atrioventricular septal defect. The recent recognition of a duplication underlying Charcot-Marie-Tooth disease (23) raises the hope that a similar duplication may be found involving chromosome 21 genes in children with isolated atrioventricular septal defect. An alternative is to seek evidence of linkage. Although collagen VI may not be a primary candidate, it may be indirectly involved in the pathogenetic processes. Howard et al. (24) found that there is an association between paternal genotype and the presence or absence of heart malformations in children with Down syndrome. Because the majority of children with Down syndrome receive their extra chromosome 21 from their mother, the inference is that trisomy 21 predisposes to heart malformation but expression is dependent in humans on a gene or genes on chromosome 21 from the other parent. Further work is needed to validate this hypothesis.

Recent developments in experimental embryology and molecular biology allow a direct approach to the identification of candidate genes by extraction of RNA from embryonic tissues leading to the creation of a library of complementary DNA fragments. In a recent report, Rezaee et al. (25) used cultured embryonic cardiocytes because the conditioned media from such cultures induce epithelial/mesenchymal transformation and it is easier to obtain good-quality RNA from cultured tissue. These investigators screened for clones containing part or all of the gene of interest using an antiserum generated against the proteins in the 100,000 kDa range.

It is likely that a very large number of genes (probably numbering in the thousands) influence early development. Furthermore, the fact that a gene is expressed in a tissue is not in itself proof of function because gene transcription may continue beyond the time of action. It is now recognized that RNA transcripts may be found in a cell where the gene has no known function. Such illegitimate transcription is exploited diagnostically by detecting the RNA transcript from the dystrophin gene responsible for Duchenne muscular dystrophy in white blood cells.

Nevertheless, demonstration that a gene is temporally and spatially expressed in the appropriate site must make the gene interesting in the search for the causes of malformation in that structure. If it can be shown that the gene maps to chromosome 21 and affects structures involved in the phenotype of Down syndrome, the case for investigation becomes even stronger.

ISOLATED ATRIOVENTRICULAR SEPTAL DEFECT

Heart malformations are usually sporadic but occasionally particular defects can be shown to be inherited as a simple Mendelian trait (26,27). Atrioventricular septal defect is associated with a 10% recurrence rate in family studies (28–30) and behaves as a simple dominant trait in some families. Figure 2 shows the most extensive pedigree published to date (31) in which isolated atrioventricular septal defect was transmitted with variable penetrance through three generations. Given the close association between atrioventricular septal defect and Down syndrome, a natural progression was to carry out linkage analysis using markers in the "Down critical region." Figure 3 shows the map location of the polymorphic markers used and Figure 4 depicts the multipoint analysis, which excludes the gene in this family from the area of the chromosome thought to be responsible for the Down phenotype. This is not too surprising given the complexity of early development. Presumably the gene is involved in the same pathway but is located on a different chromosome. Cousineau et al. (32) recently published a similar linkage analysis in a family with isolated atrioventricular septal defect and also found no evidence of linkage to chromosome 21 in the Down critical region. In one of the family members reported by Wilson et al. (31), there was coarctation in addition to atrioventricular septal defect. De Biase et al. (33) noted that atrioventricular septal defect in patients who do not have Down syndrome was frequently associated with left-sided

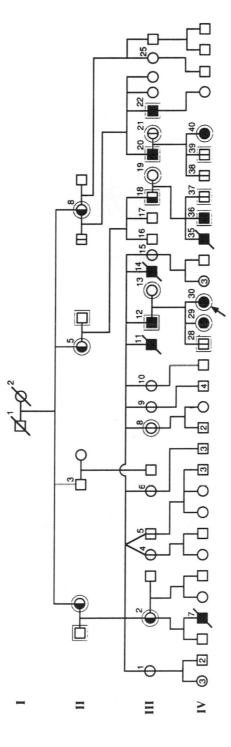

Figure 2. A large pedigree with autosomal dominant atrioventricular septal defect suitable for linkage analysis (23). ☐ indicates individuals who were not clinically examined, ◫ indicates an individual who had no clinical abnormalities on examination, ◨ represents an individual who had no abnormalities on clinical examination but who is an obligate carrier, ■ represents a family member with an atrioventricular septal defect, and ◙ indicates individuals from whom DNA samples were obtained. (From Wilson L, Curtis A, Korenberg JR, et al. A large dominant pedigree of atrioventricular septal defect: exclusion from the Down syndrome critical region on chromosome 21. *Am J Hum Genet*. 1993;53:1262–1268. Reprinted with permission of the University of Chicago Press.)

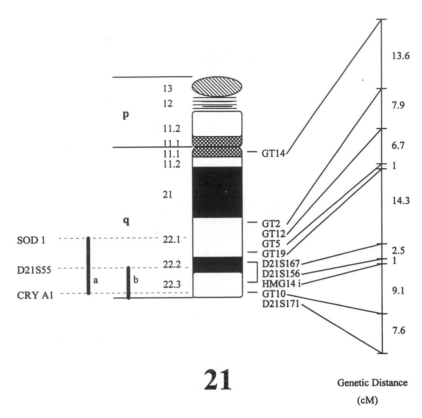

Figure 3. Polymorphic markers used in the linkage study. The distance between markers is depicted in centiMorgans on the right whereas the regions implicated in heart malformation are shown on the left. (From Wilson L, Curtis A, Korenberg JR, et al. A large dominant pedigree of atrioventricular septal defect: exclusion from the Down syndrome critical region on chromosome 21. *Am J Hum Genet*. 1993;53:1262–1268. Reprinted with permission of the University of Chicago Press.)

obstructive lesions, a feature rarely noted in children with Down syndrome that suggests a distinct embryologic mechanism (see Chapter 10).

Marino et al. (34) reported an association between atrioventricular septal defect and deletion of the short arm of chromosome 8. It is possible that identification of the gene responsible on chromosome 8 may permit the major pathway to be determined, which may then allow the chromosome 21 gene to be isolated.

CONCLUSION

The gene or genes on chromosome 21 responsible for the characteristic features of Down syndrome have not yet been identified, but it

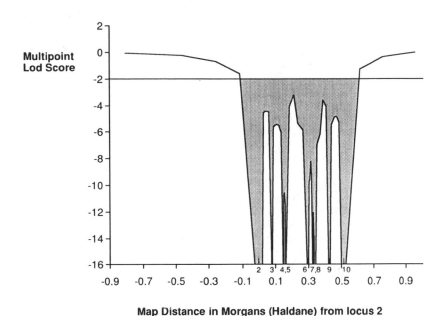

Multipoint Lod Score

Map Distance in Morgans (Haldane) from locus 2

Figure 4. Multipoint linkage analysis between marker gt2 and D21S71. The LOD score is less than −2 between these markers excluding the disease gene in this family from the critical region. (From Wilson L, Curtis A, Korenberg JR, et al. A large dominant pedigree of atrioventricular septal defect: exclusion from the Down syndrome critical region on chromosome 21. *Am J Hum Genet.* 1993;53:1262–1268. Reprinted with permission of the University of Chicago Press.)

is clear that the rapid progress toward complete mapping of chromosome 21 soon will lead to the sequencing of all expressed sequences in the critical region. When this is achieved, we will be within reach of a full understanding of the atrioventricular septal defect and an important step toward explaining how the human heart is constructed.

REFERENCES

1. Rashkind WJ. Historical aspects of congenital heart disease. *Birth Defects* (Original Article Series No. 8). 1972;1:2–8.
2. Pignatti PF, Turco AI. Tracking disease genes by reverse genetics. *J Psychiat Res.* 1992;26:287–298.
3. Stoll C, Alembik Y, Dott B, et al. Epidemiology of Down syndrome in 118,265 consecutive livebirths. *Am J Med Genet.* 1990 (suppl);7:79–83.
4. Petersen MB, Frantzen M, Antonarakis SE, et al. Comparative study of microsatellite and cytogenetic markers for detecting the origin of the nondisjoined chromosome 21 in Down syndrome. *Am J Hum Genet.* 1992;51:516–525.
5. Petersen MB, Schinzel AA, Binkert F, et al. Use of short sequence DNA polymorphism after PCR amplification to detect the parental origin of

the additional chromosome 21 in Down syndrome. *Am J Hum Genet.* 1991;48:65–71.

6. Thompson IM, Thompson DD. Male fertility and the undescended testis in Down syndrome: how to counsel parents. *Postgrad Med J.* 1988;84: 302–303.

7. Merkatz IR, Nitowski HM, Macri JN, Johnson WE. An association between low maternal serum alpha fetoprotein and fetal chromosome abnormalities. *Am J Obstet Gynecol.* 1984;148:886–891.

8. Wald NJ, Kennard A, Densem JW, Cuckle HS, Chard T, Butler L. Antenatal maternal serum screening for Down syndrome: results of a demonstration project. *BMJ.* 1992;305:391–394.

9. Spencer K, Coombs EJ, Mallard AS, Ward AM. Free beta human chorionic gonadotrophin in Down syndrome screening: a multicentre study of its role compared with other biochemical markers. *Ann Clin Biochem.* 1992;29:506–518.

10. Cuckle HS, Wald NJ, Goodburn SF, Sneddon J, Amess JAL, Carlson-Dunn S. Measurement of activity of urea resistant neutrophil alkaline phosphatase as an antenatal screening test for Down syndrome. *BMJ.* 1990;301:1024–1026.

11. Korenberg JR, Bradley C, Disteche CM. Down syndrome: molecular mapping of the congenital heart disease and duodenal stenosis. *Am J Hum Genet.* 1992;50:294–302.

12. Korenberg JR, Kawashima H, Pulst S, et al. Molecular definition of a region of chromosome 21 that causes features of the Down syndrome phenotype. *Am J Hum Genet.* 1990;47:236–246.

13. Korenberg JR, Kawashima H, Pulst SM, Allen L, Magenis E, Epstein CJ. Down syndrome: toward a molecular definition of the phenotype. *Am J Med Genet.* 1990;7:91–97.

14. Rahmani Z, Blouin JL, Creau-Goldberg N, et al. Critical role of the D21S55 region on chromosome 21 in the pathogenesis of Down syndrome. *Proc Natl Acad Sci USA.* 1989;86:5958–5962.

15. Sinet PM, Rahmani Z, Theophile D, et al. Molecular definition of 7 minimal regions on chromosome 21 involved in the pathogenesis of 23 features of Down syndrome. *Cytogenet Cell Genet.* 1991;58:2041.

16. Cox DR, Epstein CJ. Comparative gene mapping of human chromosome 21 and mouse chromosome 16. *Ann NY Acad Sci.* 1985;450: 169–177.

17. Nadau JH, Davisson MT, Doolittle DP, et al. Comparative map for mice and humans. *Mammalian Genome.* 1992;3:480–536.

18. Epstein CJ, Cox DR, Epstein LB. Mouse trisomy 16: an animal model of human trisomy 21 (Down syndrome). *Ann NY Acad Sci.* 1985;450: 157–168.

19. Epstein CJ. Mouse models for Down's syndrome and Alzheimer's disease. *Le Foundation pur letude de systeme nerveux* 1988;5:127–134.

20. Burn J, Richards SJ, Brennan P, Wyse RKH. Molecular genetic strategies on the investigation of congenital malformations. In: Clark EB, Takao H, eds. *Developmental Cardiology: Morphogenesis and Function.* Mt. Kisco, NY: Futura Publishing: 1990:557–571.

21. MacDonald G, Chu ML, Cox DR. Fine structure physical mapping of the region of mouse chromosome 10 homologous to human chromosome 21. *Genomics.* 1991;11:317–327.

22. Kurnit DM, Aldridge JF, Matsuoka R, Matthysse S. Increased adhesiveness of trisomy 21 cells and atrioventricular canal malformations in Down syndrome. A stochastic model. *Am J Med Genet.* 1985;20: 385–399.
23. Wilkie AOM. The molecular basis of genetic dominance. *J Med Genet.* 1994;31:89–98.
24. Davies GE, Howard CM, Farrer MJ, Coleman MM, Bennett LB, Cullen LM, Wyse RKH, Burn J, Williamson R, Kessling AM. Genetic variation in the COL 6A1 region is associated with congenital heart defects in trisomy 21 (Down's syndrome). *Annals Hum Genet.* 1995;59:253–269.
25. Rezaee M, Isokawa K, Halligan N, Markwald RR, Krug EL. Identification of an extracellular 130-kDa protein involved in early cardiac morphogenesis. *J Biol Chem.* 1993;268(19):14404–14411.
26. O'Nuallain S, Hall JG, Stamm SJ. Autosomal dominant inheritance of endocardial cushion defects. *Birth Defects.* 1977;13/3A:143–147.
27. Yao J, Thompson MW, Trusler GA, Trimble AS. Familial atrial septal defect of the primum type: a report of four cases in one sibship. *J Can Med Assoc.* 1968;98:218–219.
28. Sanchez-Cascos A. The recurrence risk in congenital heart disease. *Eur J Cardiol.* 1978;7:197–210.
29. Emanuel R, Somerville J, Inns A, Withers R. Evidence of congenital heart disease in the offspring of parents with atrioventricular defects. *Br Heart J.* 1983;49:144–147.
30. Digilio MC, Marino B, Cicini MP, Giannotti A, Formigari R, Dallapiccola B. Risk of congenital heart defects in relatives of patients with atrioventricular canal. *Am J Dis Child.* 1993;147:1295–1297.
31. Wilson L, Curtis A, Korenberg JR, et al. A large, dominant pedigree of atrioventricular septal defect: exclusion from the Down syndrome critical region on chromosome 21. *Am J Hum Genet.* 1993;53:1262–1268.
32. Cousineau AJ, Lauer RM, Pierpont ME, et al. Linkage analysis of autosomal dominant atrioventricular canal defects: exclusion of chromosome 21. *Hum Genet.* 1994;93:103–108.
33. De Biase L, Di Ciommo V, Ballerini L, Bevilacqua M, Marcelletti C, Marino B. Prevalence of left-sided obstructive lesions in patients with atrioventricular canal without Down's syndrome. *J Thorac Cardiovasc Surg.* 1986;91:467–472.
34. Marino B, Reale A, Giannotti A, Digilio MC, Dallapiccola B. Nonrandom association of atrioventricular canal and del(8p) syndrome. *Am J Med Genet.* 1992;42:424–427.

CHAPTER 3

MOLECULAR AND STOCHASTIC BASIS OF CONGENITAL HEART DEFECTS IN DOWN SYNDROME

Julie R. Korenberg and David M. Kurnit

DOWN SYNDROME OR TRISOMY 21 is a major cause of congenital heart disease and mental retardation and affects the welfare of over 300,000 individuals and their families in the United States alone and millions worldwide. In addition, Down syndrome is associated with a characteristic set of physical features; defects of the immune, endocrine, and gastrointestinal systems; and an increased risk of leukemia and an Alzheimer-like dementia. This chapter presents a model for isolating the genes for complete phenotypes, with particular emphasis on congenital heart disease in Down syndrome. It also reviews the role of chance or stochastic processes in devel-

This work took place in part in a SHARE's Child Disability Center and was supported by grants from the NIH (5 R29 HG00037-03 and 1 RO1 HL50025), the American Health Assistance Foundation, the American Heart Association, and the March of Dimes Birth Defects Foundation. We gratefully acknowledge the technical assistance of X.-N. Chen, S. Gerwehr, R. Gonsky, R. Schipper, and Z. Sun. Dr. Korenberg holds the Brawerman Chair of Molecular Genetics Research and Dr. Kurnit is an Investigator, Howard Hughes Medical Institute.

Considerable text used for this review was taken from References 3 and 36. We thank the *American Journal for Medical Genetics* (1985;30:385–399) and Futura Publishing Company (*Developmental Mechanisms of Heart Disease*; 1995:581–596) for permission to use this material.

opment with particular reference to the risk of congenital heart disease in Down syndrome.

FREQUENCY OF CONGENITAL
HEART DEFECTS IN DOWN SYNDROME

Down syndrome is a major cause of congenital heart defects affecting the welfare of over 300,000 individuals and their families in the United States alone. The specificity of chromosome 21 for endocardial cushion defects is illustrated by the finding that 70% of all endocardial cushion defects are associated with Down syndrome. Although a congenital heart defect is clinically present in over 40% of individuals with Down syndrome, cardiac defects are seen at autopsy in two thirds of all cases (of which nearly 70% are defects of the endocardial cushion). The majority of endocardial cushion defects found in the population as a whole are in fact those associated with Down syndrome. Although endocardial cushion defects account for at least 60% of congenital heart defects in patients with Down syndrome, they represent only 2.8% of isolated congenital heart diseases (1).

ANATOMY OF ENDOCARDIAL CUSHION DEFECTS

Endocardial cushion defect, or persistent atrioventricular canal or atrioventricular septal defect, is a malformation localized in the venous inflow region of the heart. It is a combined defect of the lower part of the interatrial septum, the ostium primum, and the upper part of the interventricular septum. It is caused by the failure of the dorsal and ventral endocardial cushions to fuse in the embryonic mesenchyma. The failure of the endocardial cushions to fuse yields a spectrum of lesions, extending from ostium primum patency with valvar anomaly to persistence of the common atrioventricular canal and membranous ventricular septal defect, all seen in Down syndrome.

STOCHASTIC FACTORS IN
DOWN SYNDROME CARDIOGENESIS

The Down Syndrome Phenotype: Increased Cellular Adhesiveness

As documented in Chapter 7, Down syndrome is strongly associated with congenital heart disease, especially with atrioventricular canal defects due to anomalies of the endocardial cushions. Spurred by these findings, we examined the adhesiveness of cardiac cushion fibroblasts. Endocardial cushion–derived tissues were isolated by dissection of the appropriate cardiac structures by Van Praagh and

Matsuoka from 20-week abortus subjects. After dissection, the tissues were explanted yielding the isolation of fibroblasts in tissue culture. Pulmonary and skin fibroblasts were isolated by mincing lung and skin tissue from these abortuses and explanting into culture. The chromosome constitutions of both experimental abortuses with trisomy 21 and control normal abortuses were confirmed by karyotype. Fibroblasts were plated at a concentration of 10^5 cells per 100-mm tissue culture dish and allowed to grow for 48 hours. The cells were resuspended to give singlets in 0.2% (wt/vol) EDTA in phosphate-buffered saline (calcium-free and magnesium-free), ph 7.4. Divalent cation–free aggregation rates were then followed by plotting the percentage of cells present in aggregates of two or more cells. We observed that cardiac cushion–derived fibroblasts from two trisomy 21 abortuses and pulmonary fibroblasts from five trisomy 21 abortuses showed significantly greater aggregation than matched control cardiac cushion–derived and pulmonary fibroblasts from eight control normal abortuses. As a further control, the low-normal rate of aggregation was observed for skin fibroblasts derived from either the experimental or the control abortuses. In summary, cardiac cushion–derived and pulmonary fibroblasts from Down syndrome subjects adhered more avidly than control normal and/or skin fibroblasts.

The Threshold Model

Based on these aggregation results, we developed computer simulations to show how a stochastic model based on the above experimental observations could describe congenital heart defects as seen in Down syndrome (2,3). Given these simulations, we showed that identical genotypes and environments may yield different results during cardiogenesis. Furthermore, we demonstrated that stochastic single-gene models describe adequately the quantitative specifications for which polygenic models were elaborated, with risk depending on the closeness and number of affected relatives (2,3) (Figure 1).

Finally, we illustrated how chance could play a significant role in cardiogenesis in particular, with extension to the general role that chance might play in development.

Epidemiology of Cardiac Septal Defects

Most congenital heart defects in persons with Down syndrome result from an atrioventricular canal defect due to abnormal outgrowth of tissues that relate to the endocardial cushions. Significant variability occurs, with a plurality of individuals with Down syndrome manifesting overt congenital heart defects. These malformations include complete, ventral (membranous-type ventricular septal defects), and

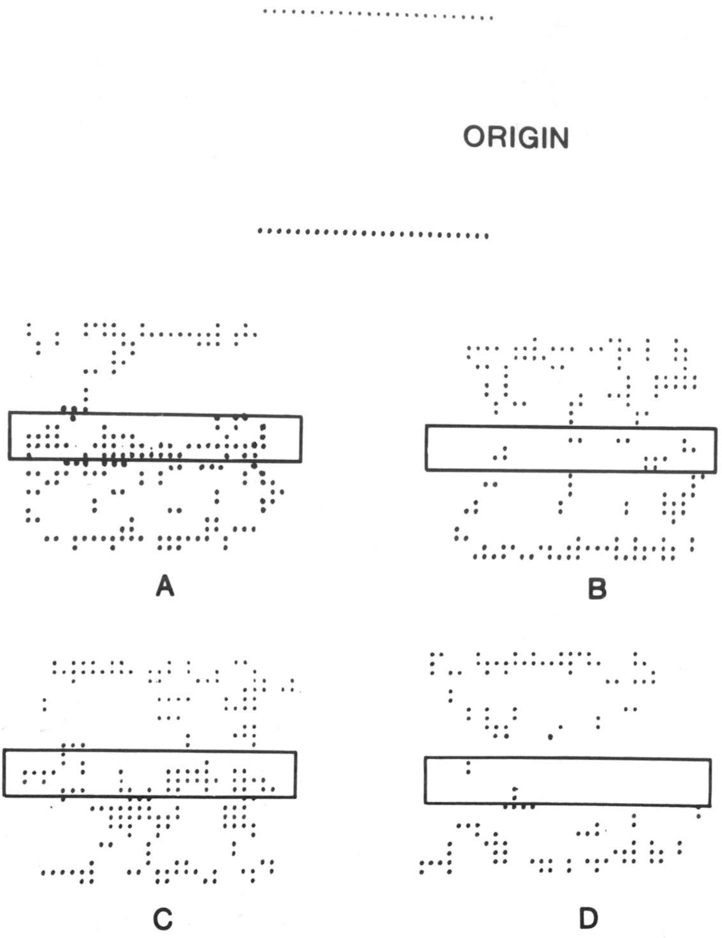

Figure 1. Threshold model for stochastic monogenic inheritance. The computer simulations that depict endocardial cushion-to-cushion fusion (2,3) were run 1,000 times apiece for a given set of parameters. The number of cells in the targeted rectangle (representing the region of cushion-to-cushion fusion) was counted at the end of each simulation, when no nonadherent cells remained. Each panel depicts the tabulation for this number of cells following multiple simulations using a given set of parameters. The abscissa gives the number of cells in the targeted rectangle and the ordinate gives the fraction of simulations using a given set of parameters that yielded that number of cells in the rectangle. The line perpendicular to the abscissa at 25 cells indicated the threshold value, below which too few cells were judged to be present to yield a normal cushion-to-cushion fusion. In the simulations the probability of migration was set at .7, the probability of division was set at .2, the probability of quiescence was set at .1. A gradient of migration was employed so that cells from the upper cushion were more likely to move downward and vice versa. In each panel a different value of adhesiveness (A) was used. In each panel, the percentage of simulations that yield abnormal simulations with less than 25 cells in the targeted rectangle is given. As the adhesiveness is increased, there is a trend that fewer cells reach the targeted rectangle, increasing the probability of an endocardial cushion defect. Because only a single parameter, adhesiveness, is varied among the panels, Figure 1 exemplifies a single-gene stochastic model. To test whether the curves in Figure 1 conformed to a normal distribution, we employed a Kolmogorov–Smirnov test (34). The curves for $A = 0.15, 0.20$ and 0.25 did not differ significantly from the natural distribution using this test ($p > .05$); the curve for $A = 0.30$ was truncated, so that application of this test was not appropriate.

dorsal (atrial septal defects) atrioventricular canal defects. Even subjects with Down syndrome who do not have a clinically significant defect may manifest a *forme fruste* characterized by enlargement of the membranous ventricular septum relative to muscularized ventricular septum (4). Discordance for congenital heart defects between monozygotic twins with Down syndrome has been noted (5). In the murine trisomy 16 for human trisomy 21, inbred trisomy 16 littermates are also discordant for congenital heart defects (6), again supporting the importance of stochastic effects.

A recent comprehensive survey (7) of the epidemiology of ventricular septal defects supported the conclusion that chance plays a major role in the etiology of ventricular septal defects in humans. Incidence rates for ventricular septal defect are similar in different races and seasons and do not correlate with maternal age, birth order, sex, or socioeconomic status. Few cases are attributable to teratogens. Although genetic factors are implicated by a recurrence risk between 1% and 5% for congenital heart defects in first-degree relatives (8), most ventricular septal defects are not associated with recognized Mendelian or chromosomal syndromes. Further support for the role of stochastic effects comes from the finding that monozygotic twins, who share identical genotypes and similar prenatal environments, show a high discordance rate for ventricular septal defect (only 2 of 26 concordant) (7).

In some cases, ventricular septal defects may occur by chance without genetic predisposition. For example, ectopia cordis (which does not show familial clustering and which is associated with heart defects including ventricular septal defects) (9) results from a developmental accident at 3 weeks' gestation (8). All of these findings indicate that both genetics and chance are causal in the etiology of cardiac septal defects.

Stochastic Single-Gene Model:
Comparison Between Observed and Predicted Data

The epidemiology of malformations not associated with recognized Mendelian syndromes has several features that must be explicable under any model purporting to explain non-Mendelian transmission. Below we detail how the stochastic single-gene model can explain these features.

In general, the recurrence risk increases with the number of affected relatives (10), with the severity of the defect in the index case, and if the index case occurs in a group (e.g., a particular sex or ethnic group) in which the malformation is less commonly seen. In the stochastic single-gene model, as in the polygenic model, such cases would likely have a more abnormal genotype whose risk curve (Figure 1) (3) is shifted further from the norm. In the stochastic single-gene model, such cases with a more abnormal genotype would correspond to homozygotes for an abnormal allele, to the more abnormal allele of a series of mutant alleles at a single locus, and/or to a single mutant gene locus associated with higher risks than other mutant loci in different families.

Single-gene Mendelian syndromes are recognized on the basis of phenotypes, which are often complex. Most such recognizable syndromes (11) consist of a constellation of features, any one of which is present in only a fraction of those with the disorder. Thus, stochastic factors operate in Mendelian malformation syndromes as well, resulting in the variability with which different features of the syndrome are found in different affected individuals, even in the same kindred in which the genetic abnormality at the affected locus is identical. In this light, Mendelian syndromes can be considered as a special case of the stochastic single-gene model. Assuming this model, Mendelian transmission of a syndrome ensues from either a high probability of manifesting one or a few traits or from moderate probabilities of manifesting any of a larger number of traits. In sum, the single-gene stochastic model can satisfy the specifications for which polygenic models were elaborated.

Role of Chance in Development

The concepts that we outline should be applicable to a wide variety of events in morphogenesis. Details of the mechanics of the model are not critical. For example, other computer simulation models (12) that made very different assumptions about how migration and adhesiveness might affect morphogenesis also yielded significant variability on a stochastic basis. Inorganic growth processes determined by surface tension and diffusion may also be simulated by an irreversible stochastic model (13). Thus, although our simulations were meant to model cardiogenesis, the concepts we outline should apply to any event in which small numbers of units interact, in probabilistic fashion, in a way that influences later masses involving larger aggregates (see Figure 3 on p. 30). Because an 8-day mouse embryo has approximately 10^4 cells (14) and our simulations involved up to 10^4 cells (3), the embryo and its constituent organs do indeed contain a sufficiently small number of cells at critical times of organogenesis.

A major concept that is evident in our simulations is that randomness evolves from *sensitive dependence on initial condition and events*. In traditional classical mechanisms, two objects that start close together and obey the same deterministic laws will remain near each other over time. In contrast, in many common dynamic systems, it is now known that however close the starting points of two objects, they may eventually be found far apart (15). Thus, even a deterministic system may behave in a "chaotic" or unpredictable way. Dynamic systems sensitive to initial conditions and/or to small perturbations early during their evolution will amplify stochastic events so that the eventual outcome may, as in our simulations, evidence randomness (15,16).

In our view, randomness is inherent in embryology, not merely an artifact of the incomplete state of our understanding of developmental processes. It is not a fundamental randomness in the quantum-mechanical sense (i.e., an uncertainty that escapes all possible reduction by measurement). If the position and characteristics of every cell in the developing embryo were known, it would be possible in principle to predict its development, and there would be no randomness in outcome. Rather, biologic uncertainty ensues from sensitivity to early perturbations: If the state of the embryonic system is described at the level of detail proper to biology, small but significant fluctuations will occur from embryo to embryo; amplification of these fluctuations yields an element of randomness in developmental outcome that cannot be escaped.

GENETIC FACTORS IN DOWN SYNDROME CARDIOGENESIS

The Pathogenetic Segment of Chromosome 21 for Congenital Heart Defects

The next step is to clone candidate genes to mediate the congenital heart defects in Down syndrome. Although Down syndrome is usually caused by the presence of an extra chromosome 21 (trisomy 21), a subset of the phenotype is caused by the presence of triplication for only parts of chromosome 21. Study of these rare individuals enables us to correlate the complex of disorders referred to as Down syndrome with triplications of particular regions of chromosome 21. The first of such studies suggested that triplication of the distal region of chromosome 21, 21q22, was sufficient to generate the recognizable features of Down syndrome, including congenital heart defects (17). The recent development of a physical molecular map of chromosome 21 (18) now allows the definition of genes for particular Down syndrome features. One approach to this combines the phenotypic information from the individuals with "partial trisomy" such as those described above with a molecular definition of their duplicated chromosomal regions. Once the molecular markers for a region are defined, the genes within it may be identified, characterized, and ultimately tested for their relationship to a given phenotype. As a first step in constructing such a "phenotypic map," a panel of 16 individuals with partial duplications of chromosome 21 was assembled and their breakpoints were established. The molecular analysis of the regions duplicated in this panel utilized a knowledge of the chromosome 21 physical map as discussed below.

Physical Map of Chromosome 21

Chromosome 21 is the smallest of human autosomes with the long arm (21q) encompassing about 40 Mb, including approximately 10^3 genes. Clones for a backbone map (with a few gaps) have been isolated in yeast artificial chromosome vectors (YACs) (19) and about 50 expressed genes have been defined, of which 25 are of known function. A summary of some of these genes is shown in Figure 2. The map of chromosome 21 includes more than 100 single-copy cloned DNA markers and more than 160 sequence tagged sites. A key point is that the physical map of chromosome 21 is sufficiently detailed to define the molecular breakpoints of most patients' duplicated regions at a resolution of 0.3–1.0 Mb.

Molecular Definition of Chromosome 21 Duplications

Two methods are used to define the regions duplicated in patients with partial aneusomy for chromosome 21. These are quantitative southern blot dosage analysis and fluorescence in situ hybridization (20). These techniques utilize a series of previously mapped chromosome 21 DNA markers to define the copy number and/or structural rearrangement characterizing the aneusomic chromosome.

Figure 3 illustrates the determination of a duplicated region using fluorescence in situ hybridization. A major advantage of this method is the ability to use DNA markers in a broad size range (1.0–650 kb) for investigation of copy number directly on metaphase chromosomes. This simultaneously produces information both on copy number and on the structural orientation of the duplicated regions, lending clues to the mechanisms that produced the chromosomal rearrangement.

**Considerations for Down
Syndrome: Phenotypic Map Construction**

The ultimate goal of constructing a phenotypic map is to define molecularly the chromosomal regions, and ultimately the genes, that are responsible for particular phenotypes. To do this, both the phenotypes and the molecular data must be well defined. Although some individuals with small duplication exist, more often the molecular data from many individuals must be combined to define small regions of

Regional Assignment of Selected Chromosome 21 Genes

Gene symbol	Marker name	Location (GDB 11/93)
ACTL5	actin-like 5	21q
APP	amyloid beta (A4) precursor protein (protease nexin-II)	21q21.2
BCEI	breast cancer, estrogen-inducible sequence	21q22.3
CBR	carbonyl reductase (NADPH)	21
CBS	cystathionine-beta-synthase	21q22.3
COL6A1, A2	collagen, type VI, alpha 1 & alpha 2	21q22.3
CRYA1	crystallin, alpha polypeptide 1	21q22.3
ERGB	avian erythroblastosis virus E26 (v-ets) oncogene related	21q22.3
ETS2	avian erythroblastosis virus E25 (v-ets) oncogene homolog 2	21q22.3
GART	phosphoribosylglycinamide formyltransferase, phosphoribosylglycinamide synthetase, phosphoribosylaminoimidazole synthetase	21q22.1
HMG14	high-mobility group protein 14	21q22.3
IFNAR	interferon, alpha; receptor	21q22.1
ITGB2	integrin, beta 2 (antigen CD18 (p95), lymphocyte function-associated antigen 1; macrophage antigen 1 (mac-1) beta subunit)	21q22.3
KCNE1	K^+ voltage-gated channel, Isk-related subfamily, member 1	21
MX1, 2	myxovirus (influenza) resistance 1 & 2, homolog of murine (interferon-inducible protein p78)	21q22.3
PFKL	phosphofructokinase, liver-type	21q22.3
RNR2	RNA, ribosomal 2	21p12
S100B	S100 protein, beta polypeptide (neural)	21q22.3
SOD1	Cu/Zn superoxide dismutase, soluble (ALS gene)	21q22.1

Figure 2. Regional assignments of selected chromosome 21 genes. The gene symbol, marker name, and location on chromosome 21 are given for gene sequences that map to chromosome 21.

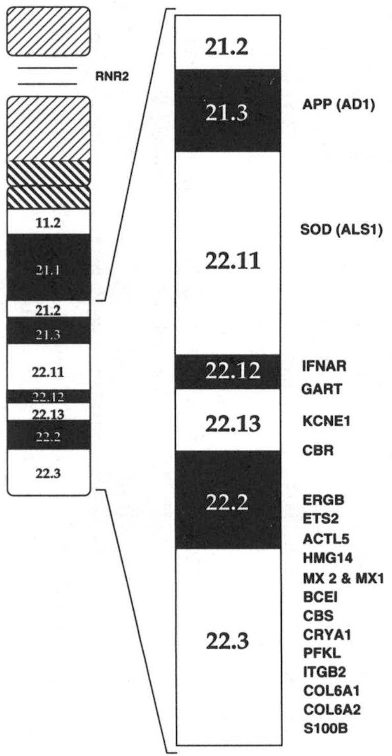

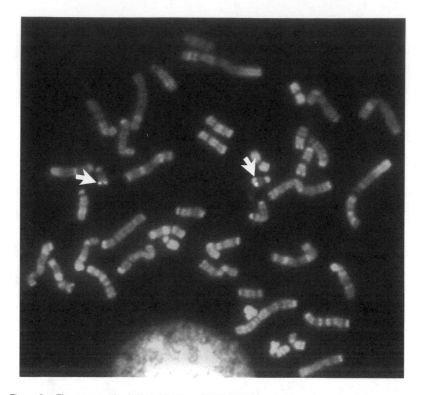

Figure 3. Fluorescence in situ hybridization of YAC 14A12 (comprising chromosome 21 markers D21S339, D21S342, and D21S159) to the chromosome 21q22.2 ⇒ p22.3 border. FITC signals, which would appear as red dots on the chromomycin/distamycin reverse-banded chromosomes, are indicated here by the arrows. (The image was captured by a Photometrics Cooled-CCD camera and Biological Detection System, Inc. [Pittsburgh] software.)

2–3 Mb that are suitable for molecular analysis. To combine data, one must consider the potential both for variability of phenotypes described previously and for multiple sites affecting a single phenotype. When a trait is caused invariably by the overexpression of a single gene or gene cluster, we may define the region containing that gene simply as the region of minimal molecular overlap of all cases exhibiting the phenotype. However, if genes in more than one region contribute significantly to the phenotype, a simple overlap procedure may erroneously define the overlap region as containing the genes. Therefore, it is important to determine which traits are caused largely by single genes or loci. To determine this one should not ask which region is responsible for a trait but rather what part of the variability of a trait is determined by the overexpression of genes in a given region.

The question may be formulated in the classical genetic terms of *penetrance* (i.e., the probability of expressing a trait given the presence of the gene responsible) and *expressivity* (i.e., the phenotypic variability of an expressed trait). It is not unreasonable to suggest that *the gene(s) in a single region are largely responsible for a given phenotype when the penetrance and the expressivity of the trait are the same in individuals with full trisomy 21 and in individuals with duplications of the single region*. Then, as we have shown, a simple overlap procedure may be used to create a phenotypic map using the molecular and clinical data from a panel of individuals with partial aneusomy. As expected, when the penetrance and expressivity suggest that a single locus is responsible for a given trait, individuals whose duplications do not include the candidate region should not express the trait of a frequency above that seen in the normal population. Based on these considerations, a phenotypic map for many of the clinically observed phenotypes of trisomy 21 emerges (Figure 4).

Congenital Heart Defect in Down Syndrome Is Caused by a Single Region on Chromosome 21

The approach to determining when a single locus is largely responsible for a trait can be illustrated by an analysis of Down syndrome and congenital heart defects. From a series of 30 cases of partial trisomy 21 reported in the literature we concluded, as reported in Epstein et al., that the distal region of 21q22 must be involved as a minimal candidate region (20). This was derived from the observation of cases with small duplications involving only this region. To estimate the proportion of Down syndrome-congenital heart defect (DS-CHD) variability that is due to a gene(s) in this region, it is necessary to determine if the risk of DS-CHD is about the same in full trisomy 21 as it is in all individuals who carry duplications for the candidate region. Furthermore, the risk of congenital heart defects to individuals *not duplicated* for this region should approximate that of the nontrisomic population. We find that 50% (9 of 18) of duplications of the distal region of 21q22 result in congenital heart defects. In addition, none of the cases (0 of 12) whose duplications do *not* include this region have congenital heart defects. Finally, similar to the phenotypic variability seen in full trisomy 21, at least one third of these congenital heart defect cases included atrioventricular septal defects, suggesting similar "expressivity."

Although ascertainment bias may inflate the total number of subjects with Down syndrome and congenital heart defects, it should not affect the determination of the region involved. In conclusion, an analysis of partial trisomy 21 from the literature suggests that dupli-

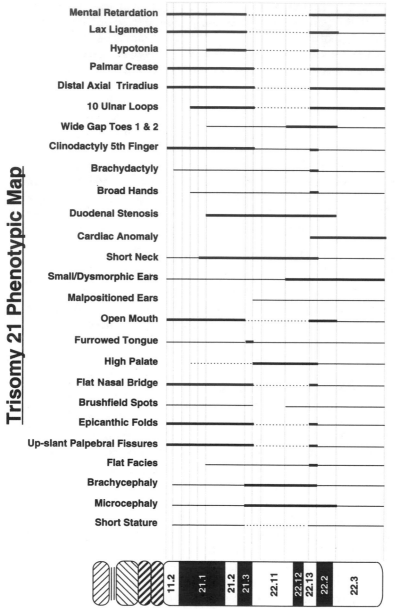

Figure 4. Trisomy 21 phenotypic map. Based on patients who show aneusomy for different portions of chromosome 21, a correlation between phenotype and genotype gives the following map for defects associated with trisomy 21.

cation of the distal region of 21q22, and not other regions, produces congenital heart defects with the same probability and phenotypic variation as full trisomy 21. In view of the specificity and spectrum of this defect in trisomy 21, we may infer the existence of a single gene or cluster in this region whose overexpression is ultimately responsible for congenital heart defects in patients with Down syndrome.

The identification of single-gene defects whose phenotype is similar to Down syndrome may also be of use. Thus, groups have now begun the investigation of families with autosomal dominant atrioventricular defects (21). If chromosome 21 markers of congenital heart defects in persons with Down syndrome are linked to the defect in these families, one may conclude that the same gene is responsible for both. However, in these cases, the family analysis excluded chromosome 21 and did not narrow the region or the candidate genes involved (21,22).

From Chromosomal Region to Gene

Once the existence of a single region has been defined for any given defect using cytogenetic or other methods, molecular markers for the region may be defined (20). Our findings indicate that the region likely to contain the genes for congenital heart defects in Down syndrome extends from D21S55 to the telomere. This region comprises approximately 9 Mb (23). Further narrowing of the region to the proximal half of this segment is suggested by combining a knowledge of the chromosome 21 physical map with data from the trisomy (Ts16) mouse. This mouse has been the animal model of Down syndrome because mouse chromosome 16 (MMU 16) shares a large homologous region with human chromosome 21 (HSA 21) (23,24). The Ts16 mice have both a high incidence and the type of congenital heart defects (6) similar to those seen in Down syndrome, suggesting that the genes in the MMU 16 regions homologous to HSA 21 may be responsible. Preliminary data indicate that this region of homology includes only the proximal half of the region duplicated in patients DUP21NA and DUP21BA—two individuals for a Down syndrome–like family with congenital heart defects (25)—and defined by D21S55 through MXI, the MX influenza virus resistance gene (23,26,27). These combined data may narrow to about 4 or 5 Mb the region of the chromosome likely to contain the gene(s) for congenital heart defects in patients with Down syndrome. A region this size contains approximately 30 expressed genes, only a subset of which should be expressed in the developing heart. This region of congenital heart defects in patients with Down syndrome is shown in Figure 5.

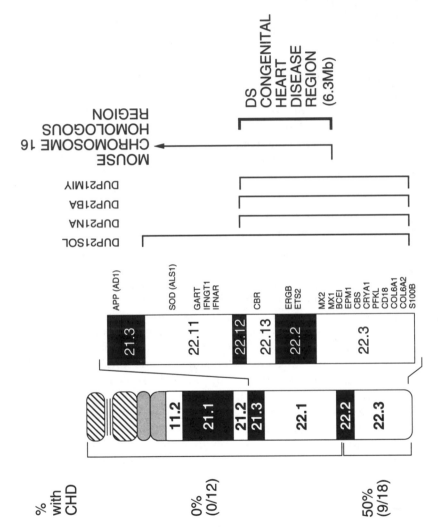

Figure 5. Region on chromosome 21 responsible for congenital heart diseases. A combination of data summarized in Figure 4 and the region responsible for congenital heart disease in mouse trisomy 16 yields a region on chromosome 21 that is likely responsible for the congenital heart diseases seen in Down syndrome.

Gene Expression and Congenital
Heart Defects in Down Syndrome

Congenital heart defects of the endocardial cushion type are due to genes expressed during the period of intense organogenesis (i.e., up to 8 weeks of development). Some of these genes may be expressed exclusively at this time. Therefore, to determine the gene responsible for some aspects of these processes it may be essential to utilize cDNA libraries constructed from this stage of development. To this end, we have used the polymerase chain reaction (PCR) to construct cDNA libraries (each with complexity = 10^6 primed both by oligo-dT and random hexamers) from a variety of human embryonic hearts and other tissues, including lung. These cDNA libraries were constructed in the phasmid λZAPII (28; Stratagene) using PCR amplification of the small amount of RNA available from an embryonic organ. Although size selection was performed to eliminate small molecules with very short cDNA inserts, the average size of inserts is 300 bp, reflecting the fact that PCR generates smaller molecules preferentially. Analogous cDNA libraries were also prepared from embryonic lungs given the abnormal aggregation phenotype we observed for pulmonary-derived fibroblasts obtained from 20-week trisomy 21 fetuses (29).

Chromosome 21 YACs (19) and derived P1 clones in the region of 21q22 responsible for congenital heart defects are fractioned and the resulting fragments subcloned as 0.5- to 2-kb fragments into the supF plasmid, pAD1 (30). pAD1-human inserts from YAC or P1 clone will be applied by an adaptation of a recombination-based assay we created (31,32) against developing heart and lung cDNA libraries (see above) to catalog the transcription pattern of these sequences in developing heart and lung. If a sequence is selected as it is transcribed in either of these tissues, counterselection isolates the corresponding gene from the cDNA library. Alternatively, other gene-hunting methodologies can be employed. Genes may also be identified from large fragment genomic pieces using procedures to selectively clone exons (33) or to select and clone cDNAs using hybridization to cloned genomic fragments fixed to magnetic beads or paper (33,34,35).

Genes so identified may then be evaluated for their potential role by sequencing, northern analysis, tissue in situ hybridization, and ultimately function in transgenic mice. Sequencing will determine the structure of the transcripts and whether the transcripts share homology with known genes. Subregional expression will be determined by labeling long cDNAs fluorescently and hybridizing in situ to sectioned cardiac and pulmonary tissue. Relevant sequences can ultimately be transfected into mice to examine the cardiac and pulmonary phenotypes that result in these transgenic mice. If positive, in addition to identifying pathogenic sequences on chromosome 21, they can be transfected into cells to determine whether these sequences are responsible for the cardiac pathology. If so, it will be of particular interest to determine whether increased aggregation correlates with pathogenicity (35,36). This will amount to a critical first step in developing strategies for intervention on behalf of affected individuals.

Implications for Clinical Genetics

This chapter presents evidence that several factors play a role in the occurrence of phenotypic differences, including inborn errors of morphogenesis. Genetics, environment, and chance all have a part in the expression of a given phenotype. The chapter emphasizes three concepts. First, chance is a significant factor in development. Second, multifactorial patterns of inheritance may be explained by single-gene models as well as by polygenic models. Third, even if it becomes feasible to predict and/or control both genotype and environment during pregnancy, birth defects will still occur as a result of chance.

REFERENCES

1. Ferencz C, Neill C, Boughman J, Rubin J, Brenner J, Perry L. Congenital cardiovascular malformations associated with chromosome abnormalities: an epidemiological study. *J Pediatr.* 1989;114:79–86.
2. Kurnit DM, Layton WM, Matthysse S. Genetics, chance, and morphogenesis. *Am J Hum Genet.* 1987;41:979–995.
3. Kurnit DM, Aldridge JF, Matsuoka R, Matthysse S. Increased adhesiveness of trisomy 21 cells and atrioventricular canal malformations in Down syndrome: a stochastic model. *Am J Med Genet.* 1985;30: 385–399.
4. Rosenquist GC, Sweeney LJ, Amsel J, McAllister HA. Enlargement of the membranous ventricular septum: an internal stigma of Down syndrome. *J Pediatr.* 1974;85:490–493.
5. Rehder H. Pathology of trisomy 21 with particular reference to persistent common atrioventricular canal of the heart. In: Burgio GR, Fraccaro F, Tiepolo L, Wolf U, eds. *Trisomy 21: An International Symposium.* Berlin: Springer-Verlag; 1981:57–73.
6. Miyabara S, Gropp A, Winking H. Trisomy 16 in the mouse fetus associated with generalized edema cardiovascular and urinary tract anomalies. *Teratology.* 1982;25:369–386.
7. Newman TB. Etiology of ventricular septal defects: an epidemiologic approach. *Pediatrics.* 1985;76:741–749.
8. Kaplan LC, Matsuoka R, Gilbert EF, Opitz JM, Kurnit DM. Ectopia cordis and cleft sternum: evidence for mechanical teratogenesis following rupture of the chorion or yolk sac. *Am J Med Genet.* 1985;21: 187–199.
9. Van Praagh R, Weinberg PM, Matsuoka R, Van Praagh S. Malpositions of the heart. In Moss AJ, Adams FH, Emmanouilides GC, eds. *Heart*

Disease in Infants, Children, and Adolescents. Baltimore: Williams and Wilkins; 1977:422–458.

10. Edwards JH. The simulation of Mendelism. *Acta Genet.* 1960;10:63–70.
11. Smith DW. *Recognizable Patterns of Human Malformation.* 3rd ed. Philadelphia: WB Saunders; 1982.
12. Fraser SE. A differential adhesion approach to the patterning of nerve connections. *Dev Biol.* 1980;79:453–464.
13. Rikvold PA. Simulations of a stochastic model for cluster growth on a square lattice. *Phys Rev.* 1982;26:647–650.
14. Ozato K, Wan Y-J, Orrison B. Mouse major histocompatibility class I gene expression begins at the midomite stage and is inducible in earlier-stage embryos by interferon. *Proc Natl Acad Sci.* 1985;82:2427–2431.
15. Ruelle D. Strange attractors. *The Mathematical Intelligencer.* 1980;2: 126–137.
16. Lorenz EN. Deterministic nonperiodic flow. *J Atmos Sci.* 1963;20: 131–141.
17. Niebuhr E. Down syndrome: the possibility of a pathogenetic segment on chromosome 21. *Humangenetik.* 1974;21:99–101.
18. Cox DR, Shimizu N. Report of the committee on the genetic constitution of chromosome 21, Human Genome Mapping II. *Cytogenet Cell Genet.* 1991;58:800–826.
19. Chumakov I, Rigault P, Guillou S, Ougen P, Bilaut A, Guasconi G, et al. Continuum of overlapping clones spanning the entire chromosome 21q. *Nature.* 1993;359:380–387.
20. Epstein C, Korenberg J, Annerén G, Antonarakis SE, Aymé S, Courchesne E, Epstein LB, Fowler A, Groner Y, Huret JL, Kemper TL, Lott IT, Lubin BH, Magenis E, Opitz JM, Patterson D, Priest JH, Pueschel SM, Rapoport ST, Sinet PM, Tanzi RE, Cruz F. Protocols to establish genotype-phenotype correlations in Down syndrome. *Am J Hum Genet.* 1991;49:207–235.
21. Wilson L, Burn J, Curtis A, Korenberg JR, Chen X-N, Chenevix-Trench G, Allen L, Goodship J. Exclusion of a defective gene within the Down syndrome critical region as the cause of atrioventricular septal defect in a large dominant pedigree. *Am J Hum Genet.* 1993;53(6):1262–1268.
22. Cousineau AJ, Lauer RM, Pierpont ME, Burns TL, Ardinger RH, Patil SR, Sheffield VC. Linkage analysis of autosomal dominant atrioventricular canal defects: exclusion of chromosome 21. *Hum Genet.* 1994; 93:103–108.
23. Gardiner K, Horisberger M, Kraus J, et al. Analysis of human chromosome 21: correlation of physical and cytogenetic maps: gene and CpG island distribution. *EMBO.* 1989;9:24–34.
24. Epstein C. *Consequences of Chromosome Imbalance: Principles, Mechanisms, and Models.* New York: Cambridge University Press; 1986.
25. Korenberg J. Down syndrome phenotypic mapping. In: Epstein C, ed. *The Morphogenesis of Down Syndrome.* New York: Wiley-Liss; 1991: 43–52.
26. Cheng S, Nadeau J, Tanzi R, et al. Comparative mapping of DNA markers from the familial Alzheimer disease and Down syndrome regions of human chromosome 21 to mouse chromosomes 16 and 17. *Proc Natl Acad Sci USA.* 1988;85:6032–6033.
27. Reeves R, Crowley M, Lorenzon N, Pavan W, Smeyne R, Golodowits D. The mouse neurological mutant weaver maps within the region of

chromosome 16 that is homologous to human chromosome 21. *Genomics.* 1989;5:522–526.

28. Short JM, Fernandez JM, Sorge JA, Huse WD. λ ZAP: a bacteriophage λ expression vector with in vivo excision properties. *Nucl Acid Res.* 1988;16:7583–7600.

29. Wright T, Orkin R, Destrempes M, Kurnit D. Increased adhesiveness of Down syndrome fetal fibroblasts in vitro. *Proc Natl Acad Sci USA.* 1984;81:2426–2430.

30. Stewart GD, Hauser MA, Kang H, McCann DP, Osemlak MM, Kurnit DM, Hanzlik A. Plasmids for recombination-based screening. *Gene.* 1991;106:97–101.

31. Kurnit DM, Seed B. Improved genetic selection for screening bacteriophage libraries by homologous recombination in vivo. *Proc Natl Acad Sci USA.* 1990;87:3166–3169.

32. Hanzlik AJ, Osemlak-Hanzlik MM, Hauser MA, Kurnit DM. A recombination-based assay demonstrates that the fragile X sequence is transcribed widely during development. *Nature Genet.* 1993;3:44–48.

33. Buckler A, Chang D, Graw S, Brook J, Haber D, Sharp P, Housman D. Exon amplification: a strategy to isolate mammalian genes based on RNA splicing. *Proc Nat Acad Sci USA.* 1991;88:4005–4009.

34. Parimoo S, Patanjali S, Shukla H, Chaplin D, Weissman S. cDNA selection: efficient PCR approach for the selection of cDNAs encoded in large chromosomal DNA fragments. *Proc Natl Acad Sci USA.* 1991;88: 9623–9627.

35. Lovett M, Kere J, Hinton L. Direct selection: a method for the isolation of cDNAs encoded by large genomic regions. *Proc Natl Acad Sci USA.* 1991;88:9628–9632.

36. Korenberg JR, Kurnit DM. Molecular and stochastic basis of congenital heart disease in Down syndrome. In: Clark EB, Markwald RR, Takao A, eds. *Developmental Mechanisms of Heart Disease.* New York: Futura; 1995:581–596.

CHAPTER 4

CONGENITAL CARDIAC MALFORMATIONS IN PATIENTS WITH DOWN SYNDROME

The Role of Atrioventricular Endocardial Cushions

Arnold C.G. Wenink
and Annemarie J.Y. Hofland

T HE DIFFERENT SPECTRUM OF CARDIAC malformations found in patients with Down syndrome and in those without this chromosomal anomaly is difficult to explain in developmental terms. Yet the differences seen are a challenge to the geneticist, and both genetic research and clinical genetics will be greatly enhanced when the key phenomenon can be described by the embryologist.

This chapter focuses on the atrioventricular septal defect (atrioventricular canal defect) that is frequently seen in Down syndrome. In an elaborate and well-documented paper, Van Praagh and collaborators (1) showed that atrioventricular septal defect may be found in syndromic and nonsyndromic forms. Among the syndromic forms, they distinguished between Down syndrome and the heterotaxy syndrome. They found that trisomic patients stand out by the absence of conotruncal malformations as double-outlet right ventricle and transposition, although Fallot's tetralogy may occur in Down syndrome.

However, the two former ventriculoarterial malformations were frequently found in patients with visceral heterotaxy.

Furthermore, in patients with atrioventricular septal defect, left ventricular outflow tract obstruction has been reported to be more frequent in the absence of Down syndrome than in its presence (2,3) (see also Chapters 7 and 10). More recently, the spectrum of ventricular septal defect has also been shown to be different in patients with and without Down syndrome (4). In that study, left ventricular outflow tract obstructions were absent in patients with Down syndrome but were frequently seen in the absence of this syndrome. Below we review the morphology of our own autopsy specimen collection in search of possible clues to the development of atrioventricular defects in persons with Down syndrome. Following that we give an account of normal cardiac embryology in terms of its relevance to the present topic.

MORPHOLOGY OF ATRIOVENTRICULAR SEPTAL DEFECT

In general, the pathology of atrioventricular septal defect can be summarized as follows (5):

1. A long and narrow left ventricular outflow tract below an unwedged aortic orifice
2. Disproportion of left ventricular inlet and outlet dimensions with a scooped inlet septum
3. A common atrioventricular junction with a five-leaflet valve, of which the left component departs completely from normal mitral morphology
4. Potential shunting at the site of the normal atrioventricular septum

A central morphologic feature is the lack of coaptation of the atrial septum and the ventricular inlet septum. Measurements have shown (5) that the length of the septum at the scoop site is shorter than the inlet length, which is the distance from the apex to the crux cordis. In addition, it was noted (5) that the inlet length is significantly shorter than the outlet length (i.e., the distance from the apex to the aortic orifice). Without further quantification, this has led to the concept of inlet septal deficiency (6,7). More recently, inlet and outlet lengths in hearts with atrioventricular septal defects were compared with the normal values (8). It was found that the inlet length in atrioventricular septal defects does not differ from that in the normal heart. Thus, any inlet septal deficiency can only reside at the site of the scoop (i.e., where the inlet septum continues into the apical trabecular septum).

The long and narrow left ventricular outflow tract may be further obstructed by abnormal papillary muscles (9,10) and by a prominent anterolateral muscle bundle (11,12). However, actual subaortic stenosis was reported to be absent in the living patient (13). The papillary muscles themselves have an abnormal position (14), which is related to the valve morphology: They are close together, particularly because of the lateral displacement of the posteromedial papillary muscle. The mural leaflet of the left (part of the) atrioventricular valve is significantly smaller than in the normal left ventricle. At the same time, the anular attachment of the valve is displaced clockwise when viewed from the apex (12).

FINDINGS

In our own autopsy collection, 69 specimens with atrioventricular septal defect were available for study. Of these, 11 were diagnosed as having the visceral heterotaxy syndrome (abnormal drainage of systemic and/or pulmonary veins, abnormal coronary sinus, atrial isomerism, right-sided aortic arch, splenic abnormalities) and 19 had Down syndrome.

To evaluate possible left ventricular abnormalities, the relative sizes of left and right ventricles were noted. Clear-cut right ventricular dominance (sometimes even with hypoplasia of the left ventricle) was seen in 3 of 11 patients with heterotaxy and in 13 of 39 patients who did not have Down syndrome, but in none of the 19 patients with Down syndrome. Obstructive anomalies of the left ventricular outflow tract were not seen in any of the heterotaxy specimens. Such lesions were noted in 20 of 39 patients without Down syndrome and in 6 of 19 with this syndrome. In many hearts, abnormalities of the papillary muscles were seen such as duplication, hypertrophy, malattachment, and additional muscles to the mural leaflet. These features were noted in more than 50% of patients without any distinction among the subgroups.

The location of the papillary muscles was identified by estimation of the angle between the main axis of a papillary muscle and the long axis of the left ventricle (i.e., the line from the arterial orifice to the ventricular apex). The anterolateral papillary muscle showed slight anterior displacement when compared to similar measurements in normal hearts, without a significant difference between patients who have Down syndrome and those who do not. The posteromedial papillary muscle showed conspicuous anterolateral displacement, with the greatest displacement found in patients without Down syndrome.

When we summarize the above findings, such left ventricular anomalies as outflow tract obstruction, ventricular hypoplasia, and abnormal papillary muscles were observed with consistent frequency in the hearts of patients who did not have Down syndrome (see also Chapters 7 and 10). The long outflow tract with unwedged aorta, the absent atrioventricular septum, the inlet–outlet disproportion, and the five-leaflet atrioventricular valve were common to all patients. In addition to the features mentioned, there were six hearts with transposition and three with double-outlet right ventricle, all of which came from the heterotaxy subgroup.

DEVELOPMENTAL CONSIDERATIONS

If one accepts that congenital malformations do not always represent the undue arrest of primitive stages (although this phenomenon does occur in teratology), there is no reason to look for any developmental stage in which the morphology of the heart would resemble that of an atrioventricular septal defect. In fact, there is no such stage.

The absence of the atrioventricular septum, which essentially is the nonfusion of the atrial septum with the ventricular inlet septum, is an important feature of atrioventricular septal defects. However, in the developmental stages in which these septal structures have not yet fused, none of the other characteristics of the malformation can be recognized. Most importantly, such embryonic hearts do not have valves (Figure 1). To block the systolic regurgitation through the atrioventricular canal, this communication between atria and ventricles is kept in check by the presence of a relatively thick wall with early differentiated myocytes for effective narrowing. Inside the canal, huge masses of endocardial cushion tissue help to stop the backflow. The ventricular cavities are heavily trabeculated and their sponge-like appearance fails to show any papillary muscles. Although it has long been thought (6,15) that the atrioventricular valves would be formed from the cushions, critical evaluation of development has shown (16–18) that the myocardial components of the heart are the more important precursors of the atrioventricular valvular apparatus. The cushions do not grow conspicuously during the period in which the muscular atrioventricular junction invaginates into the ventricular cavity to form new, flap-like structures that are the real valve primordia. At the same time, the inner trabeculated layer of the ventricular myocardium is transformed into the tension apparatus (19). The

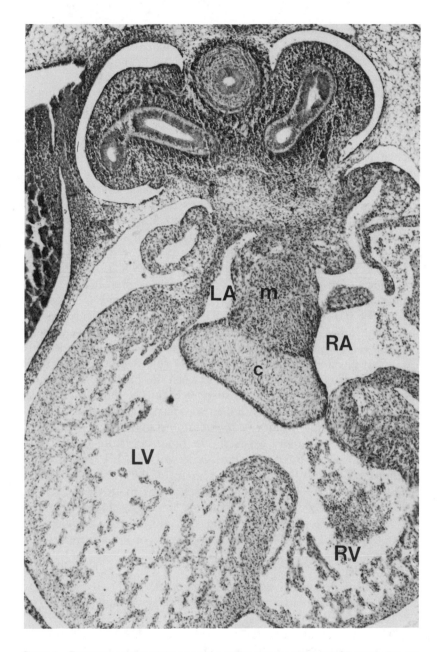

Figure 1.   Transverse section of the heart of a human embryo of 9.5-mm CR length. The atrioventrlcular canal is blocked by the inferior endocardial cushion (c). Note the mass of extracardiac connective tissue in the dorsal mesocardium (m). In the left ventricle (LV) and in the right ventricle (RV), trabeculations are numerous but no papillary muscles are seen. (LA, left atrium; RA, right atrium.)

material contribution of the endocardial cushions, as more recently advocated by Lamers et al. (20), must be small. Any abnormality of valvular morphology would therefore be better explained on the basis of the myocardial architecture of the heart.

Similar considerations are pertinent to the unwedged position of the aortic orifice in atrioventricular septal defect. This right anterior aortic displacement is not pathognomonic for atrioventricular septal defect. In Fallot's tetralogy, in which no pathology of the atrioventricular junction is found, the aortic orifice is displaced to the right and anteriorly (21). It is questionable if the aortic orifice has to change its position very much during development. Prior to fusion of the atrioventricular endocardial cushions the aorta was described as occupying its definitive position (22). Further wedging between the two atrioventricular orifices seems to depend on subsequent expansion of these as well as of the atria themselves.

As is indicated in Figure 2, expansion of the heart has important consequences for the topographic relationships. Because the atrioventricular endocardial cushions never grow beyond the absolute volume of 0.074 mm (19), their relative dimensions decrease dramatically. In fact, most of the connective tissue at the atrioventricular junction (i.e., the tissue that forms the fibrous heart skeleton [Figure 2]) is not cushion tissue but extracardiac sulcus tissue. This is the tissue that establishes a continuity between the mediastinum and the interior of the heart. As can be seen in Figure 1, this is a compact mass of tissue that forms the dorsal mesocardium and that immediately borders on the inferior endocardial cushion.

A similar continuity exists in the inner curvature of the heart (i.e., immediately posterior to the aortic orifice) (23). The superior cushion that forms the posterior border of the subaortic outflow tract has intimate relationships with extracardiac tissues at the arterial pole (Figure 2). As can be seen from the two upper diagrams in Figure 2, at least three hypothetical mechanisms can be formulated to create the characteristic "sprung" appearance of the atrioventricular junction:

1. If the two cushions do reach each other, they still may fail to fuse and further expansion of the heart may result in an abnormally posteroinferior position of the inferior cushion (15).
2. The inlet septum may fail to grow out sufficiently: It forms the septal mass at the ventricular side of the sulcus and the cushion in Figure 2 (cross-hatched area). Without doubt, the inferior cushion, which sits on the inlet septum, would never be able to reach the superior cushion (7).

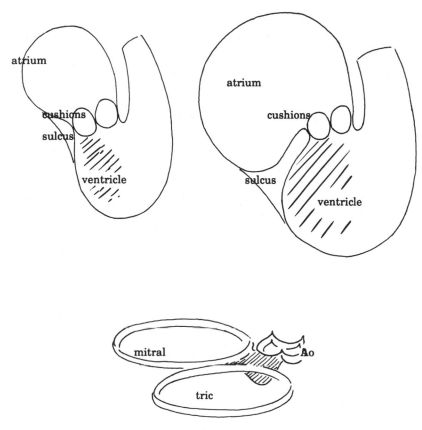

Figure 2. Diagrams to show the change of the relative dimensions of the tissues that contribute to septation. **Upper left:** Only cushion tissue is present between atrium and ventricle. The inferior cushion is positioned on top of the ventricular inlet septum (*cross-hatched*). **Upper right:** After atrial and ventricular expansion, sulcus tissue is forming the main tissue mass between atrium and ventricle. The ventricular inlet septum (*cross-hatched*) has expanded accordingly. **Bottom:** The fibrous skeleton of the mature heart. Any cushion contribution might only be expected in the area of the membranous septum (*cross-hatched*).

3. The expansion of the atrium and the ventricular inlet portion implies the incorporation of large quantities of extracardiac sulcus tissue (the dorsal mesocardium) into the heart (Figure 2). This process is not necessarily a passive one: The mesocardial tissue might, by its growth, push the inferior cushion foward. Failure of this growth might lead to a gap between the cushions. However, the way in which proliferation of the mesocardium is programmed is unknown. The factors by which the cushion tissue and the mesocardium might induce one another are largely to be elucidated.

The third hypothesis is an attractive one because it enables one to make a comparison with the developmental processes at the arterial pole. Aortopulmonary septation is effected by extracardiac tissues that are derived from the neural crest (24). When considering the complex migratory pathways of such cells, one should realize that in these very early developmental stages the distance between the branchial mesenchyme (in which the arterial pole is anchored) and the dorsal mesocardium is minimal. It may be hypothesized that influences that work primarily at the arterial pole may also be held responsible for processes concerning the inner curvature of the heart (i.e., the atrioventricular junction). Were that the case, there would be a developmental link between atrioventricular septal defect and double-outlet right ventricle, as is seen in visceral heterotaxy. In cases without ventriculoarterial lesions, as in Down syndrome, the dorsal mesocardium could be the primary target for the pathogenetic influence.

CONCLUSIONS

The contributions of extracardiac connective tissues to the heart are several. Aberrations of these contributions might lead to atrioventricular septal defects with or without ventriculoarterial malformations. The stage for these lesions is set during somewhat early development, when no valves or papillary muscles are present. These structures develop much later, and one can only speculate about the causes of their eventual variations.

Blood flow may play a role in the later morphogenetic events within the ventricles. The combination of left ventricular and mitral valve lesions with aortic stenosis and coarctation is well known and has been related to flow disturbances (25,26). If flow were that important, patients with Down syndrome (virtually without left ventricular anomalies) would need to have fairly consistent hemodynamic patterns. These patterns have to be fully elucidated, also in view of the poor postoperative hemodynamics, as were reported recently (27) (see also Chapters 13 and 14).

REFERENCES

1. Van Praagh S, Antoniadis S, Otero-Coto E, Leidenfrost R, Van Praagh R. Common atrioventricular canal with and without conotruncal malformations: an anatomic study of 251 postmortem cases. In: Nora JJ, Takao A, eds. *Congenital Heart Disease: Causes and Processes*. Mt. Kisco, NY: Futura Publishing; 1984.

2. Park SG, Mathews RA, Zuberbuhler JR, Rowe RD, Neches WH, Lennox CC. Down's syndrome with congenital heart malformation. *Am J Dis Child.* 1977;131:29–33.
3. De Biase L, Di Ciommo V, Ballerini L, Bevilacqua M, Marcelletti C, Marino B. Prevalence of left-sided obstructive lesions in patients with atrioventricular canal without Down's syndrome. *J Thorac Cardiovasc Surg.* 1986;91:467–469.
4. Marino B, Papa M, Guccione P, Corno A, Marasini M, Calabrò R. Ventricular septal defects in Down syndrome: anatomic types and associated malformations. *Am J Dis Child.* 1990;144:544–545.
5. Penkoske PA, Neches WH, Anderson RH, Zuberbuhler JR. Further observations on the morphology of atrioventricular septal defects. *J Thorac Cardiovasc Surg.* 1985;90:611–622.
6. Ugarte M, Enriquez de salamanca F, Quero M. Endocardial cushion defects: an anatomical study of 54 specimens. *Br Heart J.* 1976;38: 674–682.
7. Wenink ACG, Zevallos J-C. Developmental aspects of atrioventricular septal defects. *Int J Cardiol.* 1988;18:65–78.
8. Van Groningen JP, Hartel ME, Wenink ACG. Septal deficiency in atrioventricular septal defects. *Ann NY Acad Sci.* 1990;588:449–454.
9. Ebels T, Meijboom EJ, Anderson RH, et al. Anatomic and functional "obstruction" of the outflow tract in atrioventricular septal defects with separate valve orifices ("ostium primium atrial septal defect"): an echocardiographic study. *Am J Cardiol.* 1984;843–847.
10. Meijboom EJ, Ebels T, Anderson RH, et al. Left atrioventricular valve after surgical repair in atrioventricular septal defect with separate valve orifices ("ostium primium atrial septal defect"): an echo–Doppler study. *Am J Cardiol.* 1986;57:433.
11. Moulaert AJ, Oppenheimer-Dekker A. Anterolateral muscle bundle of the left ventricle, bulboventricular flange and subaortic stenosis. *Am J Cardiol.* 1976;37:78–81.
12. Draulans-Noe HAY, Wenink ACG. Anterolateral muscle bundle of the left ventricle in atrioventricular septal defects: left ventricular outflow tract and subaortic stenosis. *Pediatr Cardiol.* 1991;12:83–88.
13. Wenink ACG, Ottenkamp J, Guit GL, Draulans-Noe HAY, Doornbos J. Correlation of morphology of the left ventricular outflow tract with two-dimensional Doppler echocardiography and magnetic resonance imaging in atrioventricular septal defects. *Am J Cardiol.* 1989;63:1137.
14. Anderson RH, Shinebourne EA, Macartney FJ, Tynan M. Atrioventricular septal defects. In: Anderson RH, Shinebourne EA, eds, *Pediatric Cardiology.* Edinburgh: Churchill Livingstone; 1987.
15. Van Mierop LHS, Alley RD, Kausel HW, Stranahan A. The anatomy and embryology of endocardial cushion defects. *J Thorac Cardiovasc Surg.* 1962;43:71–82.
16. Wenink ACG, Gittenberger-de Groot AC. Left and right ventricular trabecular patterns. Consequence of ventricular septation and valve development. *Br Heart J.* 1982;48:462–468.
17. Wenink ACG, Gittenberger-de Groot AC. The role of atrioventricular endocardial cushion in the septation of the heart. *Int J Cardiol.* 1985; 8:25–44.

18. Wenink ACG, Gittenberger-de Groot AC. Embryology of the mitral valve. *Int J Cardiol.* 1986;11:85–98.
19. Wenink ACG. Quantitative morphology of the embryonic heart. An approach to development of the atrioventricular valves. *Anat Rec.* 1992.
20. Lamers WH, Virágh S, Wessels A, Moorman AFM, Anderson RH. Formation of the tricuspid valve in the human heart. *Circ.* 1995;91:111–121.
21. Becker AE, Connor M, Anderson RH. Tetralogy of Fallot: a morphometric and geometric study. *Am J Cardiol.* 1975;35:402–412.
22. Bartelings MM, Gittenberger-de Groot AC. The arterial orifice level in the early human embryo. *Anat Embryol.* 1988;177:537–542.
23. Van Gils FAW. The fibrous skeleton in the human heart: embryologic and pathogenetic considerations. *Virch Arch Pathol Anat Histol.* 1981; 393:61–73.
24. Beall AC, Rosenquist TH. Smooth muscle cells of neural crest origin form the aorticopulmonary septum in the avian embryo. *Anat Rec.* 1990; 226:360–366.
25. Moene RJ, Oppenheimer-Dekker A, Wenink ACG. Relation between aortic arch hypoplasia of variable severity and central muscular ventricular septal defects: emphasis on left ventricular abnormalities. *Am J Cardiol.* 1981;48:111–116.
26. Moene RJ, Oppenheimer-Dekker A, Moulaert AJ, Wenink ACG, Gittenberger-de Groot AC, Roozendaal H. The concurrence of dimensional aortic arch anomalies and abnormal left ventricular muscle bundles. *Pediatr Cardiol.* 1982;2:107–114.
27. Morris CD, Magilke D, Reller M. Down's syndrome affects results of surgical correction of complete atrioventricular canal. *Pediatr Cardiol.* 1992;13:80–84.

CHAPTER 5

DEVELOPMENTAL ASPECTS OF CONGENITAL HEART DISEASE IN CHILDREN WITH DOWN SYNDROME

Edward B. Clark

MOST CHILDREN WITH DOWN SYNDROME have an abnormal cardiovascular system. Approximately 50% have structural defects including atrioventricular canal defects. The remaining infants have more subtle abnormalities of cardiac morphology and cardiovascular function. A little-studied aspect of cardiovascular disease in Down syndrome is the functional alterations that affect embryonic and fetal development and may contribute to the high frequency of spontaneous abortion. The heart is the first functioning organ and the only one required for the continuation of in utero development. The influence of trisomy 21 on fetal outcome likely relates to the adequacy of the malformed cardiovascular system.

Because we have focused on the structural defects requiring surgical repair or leading to fixed pulmonary vascular obstructive disease in the past, more subtle structural and functional abnormalities may have been overlooked. In a morphologic study of hearts from patients with Down syndrome who do not have congenital cardiovascular abnormalities, Rosenquist found major deviations from normal hearts (1). The membranous interventricular septum was markedly enlarged (also see Chapters 10 and 12). The placenta is small compared to the fetus, and a frequent abnormality is cystic hygroma or other abnormality of the lymphatic system (2). Thus, most if not all patients with

Down syndrome have fundamental abnormalities of cardiovascular morphology.

Functional changes likely accompany these morphologic changes. In experimental studies, the initial teratogenic effect is an alteration in function that precedes an alteration in morphology. The functional effects of the trisomic cardiovascular system during fetal development are largely unexplored. Yet these functional changes likely affect outcome and determine which embryo or fetus will survive to term. The evidence to support this view comes in part from an analysis of fetal outcome following the in utero diagnosis of Down syndrome.

FETAL ECHOCARDIOGRAPHY

The developmental outcome of fetuses with Down syndrome is only now becoming clear as fetal echocardiographers follow the course of such fetuses. The combination of high-risk screening by maternal age and alpha-fetoprotein levels and confirmation by amniocentesis and karyotype have permitted prospective evaluation of the outcome of fetuses with Down syndrome. In 1983 clinicians began to monitor the outcome of pregnancy by serial assessment of growth and structure through obstetric and cardiac ultrasound (3–5). Thus, we are beginning to understand the additional factors involved in the primary cardiac abnormality and the extraordinarily high prevalence of fetal demise.

The growth pattern of fetuses with trisomy 21 is abnormal compared to that of fetuses without chromosomal aberrations. Whereas there were no differences between the biparietal diameter, head circumference, or abdominal circumference, femur length in fetuses with Down syndrome was shorter than that in fetuses with normal chromosomes (6).

Early in this experience it was recognized that the major congenital cardiovascular defect (i.e., complete atrioventricular canal) could be identified in the four-chamber view of the heart. In a study at Johns Hopkins Hospital, 20 of 300 fetuses were noted to have a congenital cardiovascular defect. When a fetus was referred for fetal echocardiography on the basis of an abnormal four-chamber view, 50% had an abnormality (7). Only 2 of the 20 infants with a variety of cardiac defects were alive and well (8). Sharland and colleagues found that 33% of fetuses with trisomy 21 died in utero (5). Among our 5 fetuses with trisomy 21, 1 died in utero.

MORPHOGENESIS AND FUNCTION

A functioning cardiovascular system is necessary for fetal survival. The contribution of the underlying cardiovascular abnormalities to the outcome is likely related to inadequate fetal cardiovascular function including arrhythmias and abnormal cardiac output. Associated abnormalities, including cystic hygroma, ascites, and pericardial effusion, may be manifestations of congestive heart failure. In the chick embryo, the developmental biology of atrioventricular septation involves the interaction of adheron-like molecular complexes and the endothelium overlying the endocardial cushions (9). Endothelial cells transform into mesenchymal tissue as these cells migrate into the myocardial basement membrane (i.e., the cardiac jelly). This process is integral to the adhesion of the endocardial cushions and the division of the atrioventricular orifice.

The lymphatic circulation is likely fundamentally abnormal among many fetuses with Down syndrome. Little is known about the lymphatic circulation during normal cardiovascular development. However, abnormalities of lymphatic flow are implicated in the pathogenesis of heart defects in monosomy 45 XO (10). Alterations in lymphatic pressure may alter blood flow, which in turn alters morphogenesis. Miyabara recently analyzed three fetuses with cystic hygroma and trisomy 21 who had lymphatic abnormalities in the absence of cardiovascular defects (2). Subtle changes in the lymphatic structure may alter formation of the coronary vascular bed and the myocardium.

There is little information available on associated defects among fetuses with Down syndrome who do not survive. For example, the character of the coronary artery bed has not been studied sequentially in a manner than can distinguish subtle abnormalities that influence ventricular function. One of the critical transitions in cardiovascular development occurs from a trabeculated ventricle to a compact myocardium with a well-established coronary artery system. There are other changes in the fetal myocardium that may be relevant. The immature myocardium has less functional reserve than the mature heart. Studies in the chick embryo, fetal lamb, and neonatal rabbit show that there are fewer contractile elements and mitochondria in the immature myocardium. The nature of calcium handling and activation contraction coupling is unknown in the myocardium of fetuses with Down syndrome.

The functional integration of the heart is in large part determined by the extracellular integrins that connect the myocytes in the warp and woof of the myocardium (11). Although the growth factors have been implicated in the process of atrioventricular septation, little is known about growth control in the formation of the myocardium. The ultrastructure of the myocardium in embryos or fetuses with Down syndrome is not available in the literature.

The automatic nervous system is integral to the precise regulation of the cardiovascular system in terms of matching cardiac output to the functional demands of the body. Although studies in older patients with Down syndrome failed to identify abnormalities by crude pressor tests, subtle defects may underlie abnormalities in cardiovascular control contributing to instability and disease.

A relatively precise measure for the clinical assessment of fetal cardiovascular function may soon become available. Current measures, including peak velocity index and wall motion, are still in development but are being carried out in some centers (12,13). However, the embryonic and fetal hearts are regulated precisely throughout the process of growth morphogenesis and function (14). New measurements that are sensitive to the regulatory cycle will likely define previously unrecognized defects in the feedback control.

Progress in the understanding of these obscure yet essential aspects of cardiovascular development in Down syndrome will come from two fronts. The first is the intensive analysis of fetuses with Down syndrome using ultrasound and Doppler techniques. The second is the sequential structural and functional analysis of normal and trisomy model of Down syndrome (15). The new information will define the mechanisms that determine growth morphogenesis and function during the critical process of cardiovascular development.

REFERENCES

1. Rosenquist GC, Sweeney LJ, Amsel J, McAllister HA. Enlargement of the membranous ventricular septum: an internal stigma of Down's syndrome. *J Pediatr.* 1974;85:490–493.
2. Miyabara S, Sugihara H, Maihara N, et al. Significance of cardiovascular malformations in cystic hygroma: a new interpretation of the pathogenesis. *Am J Med Genet.* 1989;34:489–501.
3. Coerdt W, Rehder H, Gebauer HJ, et al. Cardiac defects in chromosomally abnormal human embryos of 10–14 weeks. *Prenat Diag.* 1988; 8:647–659.
4. Gembruch U, Knopfle G, Chatterjee M, et al. Prenatal diagnosis of atrioventricular canal malformation with up to date echocardiographic technology: report of 14 cases. *Am Heart J.* 1991;121:1489–1497.
5. Sharland GK, Lockhart SM, Chita SK, Allan LD. Factors influencing the outcome of congenital heart disease detected prenatally. *Arch Dis Child.* 1990;65:284–287.

6. Dicke JM, Crane JP. Sonographic recognition of major malformations and aberrant fetal growth in trisomic fetuses. *J Ultrasound Med.* 1991; 10:433–438.
7. Lockwood CJ, Lynch L, Berkowitz RL. Ultrasonographic screening for the Down syndrome fetus. *Am J Obstet Gynecol.* 1991;165:349–392.
8. Callan NA, Maggio M, Steger S, Kan JS. Fetal echocardiography: indications for referral, prenatal diagnostic and outcomes. *Am J Perinatol.* 1991;8:390–394.
9. Markwald RR, Mjaatvetd CH, Krug EL. Induction of endocardial cushion tissue formation by adheron-like molecular complexes derived from the myocardial basement membrane. In: Clark EB, Takao A, eds. *Developmental Cardiology: Morphogenesis and Function.* Mt. Kisco, NY: Futura Publishing; 1990:191–204.
10. Lacro RV, Jones KL, Benirschke K. Coarctation of the aorta in Turner syndrome: a pathologic study of fetuses with nuchal cystic hygroma, hydrops fetalis, and female genitalia. *Pediatrics.* 1988;81:445–451.
11. Borg TK, Xuehui M, Hienski L, Vinson N, Terracio L. The role of the extracellular matrix on myofibrillogenesis in vitro. In: Clark EB, Takao A, eds. *Developmental Cardiology: Morphogenesis and Function.* Mt. Kisco, NY: Futura Publishing; 1990:175–191.
12. Groenenberg IAL, Wladimiroff JW, Hop WCJ. Fetal cardiac and peripheral arterial flow velocity waveforms in intrauterine growth retardation. *Circulation.* 1989;80:1711–1717.
13. Van der Mooren K, Barendregt LG, Wladimiroff JW. Fetal atrioventricular and outflow tract flow velocity waveforms during normal second half of pregnancy. *Am J Obstet Gynecol.* 1991;165:668–674.
14. Clark EB. Growth, morphogenesis and function: the dynamics of cardiac development. In: Moller JH, Neal W, Lock J, eds. *Fetal, Neonatal and Infant Heart Disease.* New York: Appleton-Century-Crofts; 1990: 3–23.
15. Miyabara S. Cardiovascular malformations of mouse trisomy 16: pathogenic evaluation as an animal model for human trisomy 21. In: Clark EB, Takao A, eds. *Developmental Cardiology: Morphogenesis and Function.* Mt. Kisco, NY: Futura Publishing; 1990:191–204.

CHAPTER 6

GENESIS OF CARDIOVASCULAR ANOMALIES IN MURINE TRISOMY 16

Carol Bacchus and Werner Buselmaier

SINCE THE EARLY 1980s, an animal model for human Down syndrome has been available that allows the investigation of chromosome triplication and the resulting implications in ontogeny. The murine trisomy 16 has been demonstrated in many reports as a valid model system for humans (1–3). The phenotypic similarity between murine trisomy 16 and human trisomy 21 is genetically based on the synteny of 11 genes and anonymous DNA sequences located on both the mouse and human chromosome. Of these, the genes App (amyloid precursor protein), Sod-1 (copper/zinc superoxide dismutase), Prgs (phosphoribosylglycineamide synthetase), Ifrc (α- and β-interferon receptor), Mx-1 and Mx-2 (interferon-induced influenza resistance), Ets-1 (protooncogene), and some random human DNA sequences (D21S16h, D21S52h, D21S58h) are located both in the supposed Down syndrome–specific 21q21>ter region of human chromosome 21 and on the c>ter part of mouse chromosome 16 (Figure 1) (4–10). The supposed Down syndrome region also includes a number of loci that have been localized on murine chromosome 17 and chromosome 10 (11–14), but nevertheless studies in trisomy 16 mice can help to characterize the effects of gene dosage and gene expression on organ morphogenesis and differentiation (15).

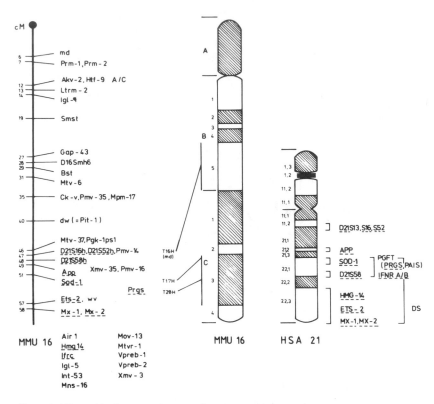

Figure 1. Recombination map of mouse chromosome 16 (MMU16) in cM, cytological map of MMU16, and cytological map of human chromosome 21 (HSA21).

Although murine trisomy 16 is not viable beyond term, many phenotypic features specific to the trisomic state, including lagophthalmos, subcutaneous edema, skeletal malformations, abnormalities of the cardiovascular system, and functional defects of the nervous and hematopoietic system, have been described in fetuses (1,2,16–19). Many of these features are also known to occur in human Down syndrome. However, in spite of extensive research work, the pathogenetic mechanisms of aneuploidy have scarcely been elucidated. Here the murine animal model provides a helpful tool with which the genesis of complex organ defects can be followed under trisomic conditions during embryogenesis.

This chapter gives a review of the cardiovascular abnormalities seen in trisomy 16 fetuses and attempts to provide a pathogenetic evaluation of trisomy 16–specific observations.

METHODS

The experimental generation of murine trisomies can be easily accomplished by mating mice carrying Robertsonian translocation chromosomes to normal diploid laboratory mouse strains. Figure 2 demonstrates the production of a murine trisomy by using males doubly heterozygous for two Robertsonian translocation chromosomes. Both metacentric chromosomes have a monobrachial homology for the chromosome to be triplicated.

The partially homologous translocation chromosomes form quadrivalents together with the corresponding acrocentric chromosomes during meiotic prophase I, which is followed by malsegregation of the homologous chromosomes. The resulting zygote is either concurrently monosomic and trisomic for the chromosomes involved in the translocation, or monosomic and/or trisomic for the chromosome involved in both Robertsonian translocations; or, finally, the resulting zygote can be disomic but carrying at least one Robertsonian chromosome. This breeding scheme was anticipated by Gropp and co-workers (20) and is generally used for the production of mouse trisomies. The induction of specific trisomies is dependent only on the combination of double heterozygotes used for breeding.

In our laboratory, we used males doubly heterozygous for the Robertsonian translocation chromosomes Rb (11.16) and Rb (16.17) and crossed these with normal C3H/HeJ females. Only disomic conceptuses and those trisomic for chromosome 16 were able to survive to term. The trisomic fetuses can be readily identified by the presence of two Robertsonian chromosomes, Rb (11.16) and Rb (16.17), plus 37 acrocentric chromosomes including the maternal chromosome 16 (Figure 3). In contrast, the disomic littermates that survived to term have only one metacentric translocation chromosome, either Rb (11.16) or Rb (16.17). However, the identification of trisomy 16 fe-

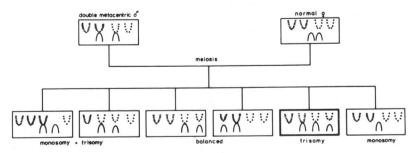

Figure 2. Breeding scheme with Robertsonian translocation chromosomes.

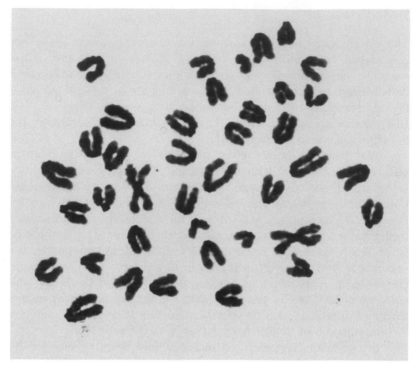

Figure 3. Karyotype of a trisomy 16 mouse fetus with two translocation chromosomes Rb (11.16) and Rb (16.17).

tuses can also be based solely on phenotypic criteria. For example, the presence of a generalized edema is a reliable morphologic marker for murine trisomy 16 with a sensitivity of 91% (16).

We assessed a total of 109 trisomy 16 fetuses on Days 18–20 of gestation (day of vaginal plug detection was designated Day 1 of gestation) for cardiovascular abnormalities. The examination was performed in the native state after shock-freezing and storage at 4°C overnight. The thorax was opened wide on one side, and the thymus was inspected and then removed to expose the heart and the great vessels. After morphologic examination of the developing cardiovascular system, the heart was opened by inserting a scissor blade from the left ventricle into the aorta, after which the ventral wall of the left ventricle was opened and the pulmonary artery severed. This procedure completely exposed the ventricular septum and allowed the detection of septal defects (16).

FINDINGS

Our results indicated that trisomy of chromosome 16 produced severe cardiac lesions and heart vessel abnormalities in 91.7% of all genetically affected fetuses. Although the phenotype did not mimic the human type of defects in all details, the frequency of malformation and the consistent pattern of observed abnormalities permitted the hypothesizing of pathogenetic mechanisms. Defects of the heart and/or the great vessels were observed in 100 of 109 trisomic fetuses (91.7%). The anomalies detected were mainly hypoplasia of the aortic arch, situs inversus or interruption of the aortic arch, and/or aplasia of the pulmonary arteries. Other anomalies, such as abnormal insertion of the pulmonary artery into the ascending aorta (truncus arteriosus), an arteria subclavia luxoria (aberrant subclavian artery), abnormal course of the aortic arch, and ventricular septal defects, occurred at a reduced frequency (Table 1).

The pattern of anomalies found in the trisomic mouse can be classified according to different criteria. Using the Rathke-type diagram (21) of the embryonic arch system, which places emphasis on vascular anomalies and assigns secondary importance to cardiac defects (Figures 4 and 5), one can differentiate among three basic types of vascular malformations: a Type L, in which the blood flowing caudally from the heart passes through part of the aortic arch system as in the normal situs; a Type R, in which parts of the right aortic arch system serve the same purpose corresponding to a mirror image of the normal configuration; and a symmetric Type S, characterized by the formation of a fourth aortic arch on both the left and right sides (double aortic arch). The latter type was seen in only one trisomic specimen.

Practically all vascular anomalies that we found can be classified with reference to these three basic types in the Rathke-type diagram, which assumes the existence of vestigial fifth arches. The aortic arch affected (IV, V, or VI) was an additional aid to the classification. In most cases the fourth (aortic) and sixth (pulmonary) arches exhibited anomalies. The least significant variation is probably the arteria subclavia lusoria (22), which had the standard form of a subclavian artery originating from the descending aorta (Figure 4: L-IV1a, R-IV1a) in both the L and the R type of system. Next to this type of an arteria subclavia lusoria, variations in which the subclavian artery terminated in the third, fifth, or sixth aortic arch (Figure 4: R-VI4, R-V1a, R-VI2a) were also observed. An arteria subclavia lusoria is regarded to be a variation without serious functional consequences because it is

Table 1. Cardiovascular anomalies in fetuses with trisomy 16

Location of arch	Abnormal arch no.	Type	Finding	No. of Cases (total)	Subtypes
Left	IV	1a, b	Ventricular-septum defect (VSD)[a]	8	3
			Arteria subclavia lusoria		2
			Truncus brachiocephalicus short[a]		3
		1	Aorta transversa runs dorsal to trachea and esophagus[a]	7	2
		a	Arteria subclavia lusoria		2
		a	Truncus brachiocephalicus short or missing[a]		3
		2	Hypoplasia of aortic arch, VSD	19	11
			Aortic arch runs dorsal to trachea and esophagus[a]		2
		a	Arteria subclavia lusoria		3
		a	Truncus brachiocephalicus missing[a]		1
			No VSD		2
		3	Aplasia of aortic arch, VSD	26	19
			Arteria pulmonalis runs dorsal to trachea and esophagus[a]		1
		a	Arteria subclavia lusoria		6
	V	1	Insertion of ductus arteriosus too far proximal	8	3
		a	Aorta transversa runs dorsal to trachea and esophagus[a]		4
		a	Arteria subclavia lusoria		1
	VI	2	Hypoplasia of Arteria pulmonalis, VSD, Truncus brachiocephalicus missing, elongated conus	7	
Symmetric arch	IV		Two symmetric aortic arches	1	
Right	IV	1	Aortic arch right-sided without further pathology	13	4
		a	Arteria subclavia lusoria		1
		2	Hypoplasia of aortic arch, VSD		4
		a	Arteria subclavia lusoria		1
		3	Aplasia of aortic arch, VSD		3
	V	1	Connection between left arteria carotis and left arteria subclavia	3	1
		a	Arteria subclavia lusoria, hypoplasia of aorta transversa, VSD		2
	VI	2	Hypoplasia of arteria pulmonalis, VSD	4	1
		3	Aplasia of arteria pulmonalis, VSD		2
		a	Arteria subclavia lusoria		1

From Bacchus C, Sterz H, Buselmaier W, Sahai S, & Winking H. (1987). Genesis and systematization of cardiovascular anomalies and analysis of skeletal malformations in murine trisomy 16 and 19. Two animal models for human trisomies. Hum Genet. 1987;77:12–22. Reprinted by permission.

[a]Not shown in Figure 4.

60

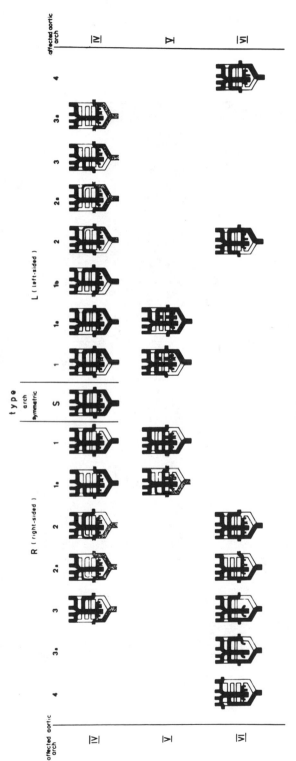

Figure 4. Rathke-type diagrams showing the variability of cardiovascular anomalies in trisomy 16 fetuses. The types VI₄ (R and L) belong to an experiment in which NMRI females were mated instead of C3H/HeJ. They are included in the scheme in order to complete the spectrum of cardiovascular anomalies encountered in trisomy 16 fetuses but are not listed in Table 1. (1 = normal; 2 = hypoplasia of arch; 3 = aplasia of arch; 4 = aplasia of ductus arteriosus Botalli; a, b = one of the possible forms of arteria subclavia lusoria; IV = prodromal aorta; V = vestigial fifth arch; VI = prodromal arteria pulmonalis.)

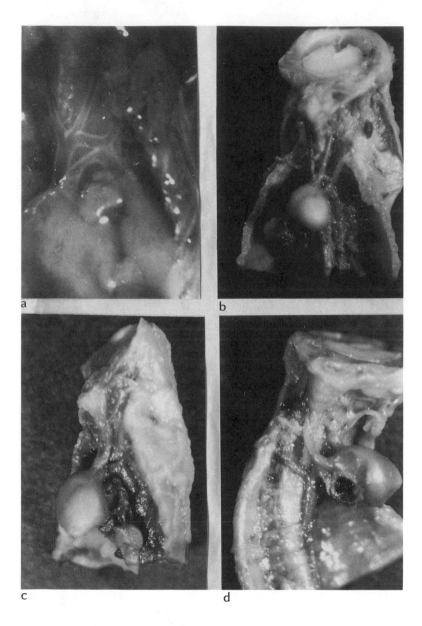

Figure 5. Ventral aspect of the cardiovascular system in situ of 20-day-old mouse fetuses. a) normal situs; b) hypoplasia of left IV aortic arch; c) aplasia of left IV aortic arch; d) arteria subclavia lusoria. (a = unfixed specimen; b–d = specimen fixed in Bouin's fluid.)

a sporadic finding in both humans and animals. Nonetheless, it can also be seen as an initial indicator of a trisomy 16–specific anomaly.

The next malformation, which occurred very frequently, was hypoplasia of the fourth aortic arch with a transfer of its function to the sixth aortic arch (Figure 4: L-IV2, R-IV2, R-V1a) and thus to the pulmonary artery, whereby the ductus arteriosus must inevitably become an integral part of the caudal circulatory system after birth. Due to partial or total obstruction of the fourth aortic arch in this anomaly, a ventricular septal defect is essential for intrauterine survival. This was regularly seen in this type of anomaly. Because this defect is not compatible with the onset of lung breathing, it is considered to be one of the causes of death during the perinatal period.

On a scale of increasingly severe vascular malformations, hypoplasia of the fourth aortic arch is logically followed by interruption of the fourth aortic arch, which we found in anomalies of types L and R-IV3 (Figure 4).

The next most severe forms were hypoplasia and interruption of the sixth aortic arch (Figure 4: L-VI2, R-VI2, R-VI3), which entailed a corresponding transfer of function to the fourth aortic arch, partly with obvious hypertrophy of an ascending aorta overriding a ventricular septal defect. The cases that we designated as R-V1 (Figure 4) were unusual defects that were observed only in Type R anomalies. In our opinion, they represent an aberrant form of the pulmonary artery where use is made of the fifth aortic arch. Our diagnosis is based on the position of the right subclavian artery, which joins the descending arch distal to the junction of aorta and pulmonary artery. The pulmonary artery most likely utilizes the fifth aortic arch. In both cases, we also found other vascular defects: in Case R-VIa, the left subclavian artery took the shorter route via the fifth aortic arch, whereas in Case R-V1 a ring was formed via a vestigial connection (embryonal dorsal aorta) between the left carotid and left subclavian arteries. Individual fetuses exhibited nearly parallel ascending aorta and pulmonary arteries with too proximal a junction of the ductus arteriosus into the aorta. This situation is not as easily classified as most other anomalies. According to Binder (21), it could represent a persisting fifth aortic arch or a sixth aortic arch beginning too proximally with a concomitant anomaly of the septum between the aorta and pulmonary artery. In Figure 4, we associated these findings with anomalies of the fifth aortic arch (Figure 4: L-V1, L-V1a).

The spectrum of cardiovascular anomalies that we encountered is described in detail in Table 1 and shown in the schematic diagram of Figure 4. In our attempt to set up a simplified classification of these anomalies, we had to compromise on the graphic presentation of certain features for practical reasons. For example, the hypothetical sixth aortic arches in malformations of Types VI3 and VI3a have been omitted in the diagrams.

A number of other vascular anomalies appeared together with the above-mentioned abnormalities but were omitted from Table 1 for the sake of clarity. These included the location of individual vessels (fourth aortic arch, right subclavian artery) behind the trachea and esophagus, and shortened brachiocephalic trunks. The ventricular septal defects ranged from a nearly absent septum to small defects located directly under the semilunar valves.

Apart from some of the above-mentioned anomalies of the cardio-vascular system, 60% of all trisomic fetuses also exhibited thymus dysplasia. In the majority of cases, the thymus consisted of two separate egg-shaped anlagen lying side by side (Figure 6). However, asymmetric hypoplasia and complete aplasia of one lobe were also observed. This finding was not unexpected as evidenced by Epstein's (1) report of hypoplasia of the thymus in trisomy 16 mice. Epstein concluded that thymic abnormalities are the result of a deficiency of prothymocytes or a defective migration of precursor cells into the primitive thymus.

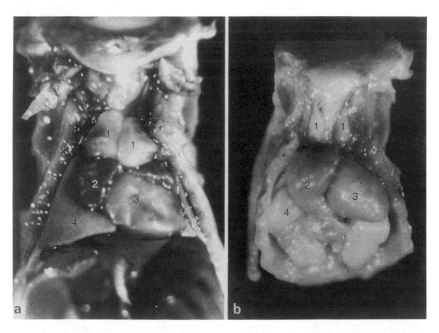

Figure 6. Ventral aspect of thoracic organs in situ of 20-day-old mouse fetuses. a = Control specimen; b = trisomy 16 fetus with hypoplasia of the thymus (1 = thymus; 2 = right atrium; 3 = heart; 4 = lungs).

The concomitant presence of thymus and cardiovascular anomalies implicates a pathogenetic mechanism that primarily affects the region of migrating cranial neural crest cells into the aortic sac. This hypothesis is also supported by the close phenotypic relationship of the trisomy 16 pathology and pharyngeal pouch abnormalities (23). In humans, analogous malformation patterns have also been associated with the DiGeorge syndrome. Although we have little information about which gene products are available in excess or in altered quantities in mouse trisomy 16 and about which regulatory mechanisms are modified in the trisomic state, we must consider the influence of migrating neural crest cells and their timed contact with specific organ buds during ontogeny (24,25) as a possible factor of developmental disruption. Neural crest migration commences on Days 7–9 of gestation in mice. If migration is triggered or adversely affected by gene expression, one would expect that the responsible genes are switched at latest on Day 7 of gestation. Moreover, to induce aortic arch malformation, gene activity would have to operate on approximately Day 10.5 of gestation (26).

In a recent survey of developmental cardiology in mouse trisomy 16, Miyabara (18) came to similar conclusions after both morphologic-histologic and scanning electron microscopy examinations of affected trisomic hearts and vessels. The survey comprised 118 trisomic specimens from five different crossings. For the majority of fetuses, a common atrioventricular canal was observed (104 cases). Among findings of the conotruncal region, double-outlet right ventricle (66 specimens), persistent truncus arteriosus (33 cases), and overriding aorta (14 cases) were observed. In all cases, a large ventricular septal defect was most apparent below the conus. Finally, 76 of all examined trisomic fetuses exhibited anomalies of the aortic arch. These were described as right-sided aortic arch, aberrant subclavian arteries, interruption of aortic arch, coarctation of aortic arch, and double aortic arch. The prevalence of specific findings was dependent on the background of the strains used. Nonetheless, Miyabara's findings (18) were well in line with the results of our investigation described above. Moreover, thymus hypoplasia was seen in every trisomic specimen. Miyabara (18) concluded that the primary insult in the pathogenesis of common atrioventricular canal was the failure of the superior and inferior endocardial cushions to fuse. This was also suggested by Van Mierop (27). The lacking fusion of the endocardial cushions in the trisomic atrioventricular canal was thought to be caused by the hypoplastic development of the endocardial cushions via delayed appearance and abnormal migration of mesenchymal cells after the 11th day of pregnancy (18). Concerning the development of aortic arch anomalies, Miyabara supported the pathognomonic appearance of aortic arch alteration and thymus hypoplasia, and the relationship to pharyneal pouch abnormalities. Similar cardiovascular findings have also been described by Pexieder et al. (28). The results were obtained only after examination of a small number of trisomic fetuses.

CONCLUSIONS

From the results of our animal experimentation, it can be concluded that the pathogenesis of murine trisomy 16–specific cardiovascular abnormalities must follow similar mechanisms operant in pharyngeal anomalies, such as in DiGeorge syndrome. Such mechanisms most likely also apply for human Down syndrome because similar cardiovascular malformations are observed in human trisomy 21 (18,29). Even if the cardiovascular defects in murine trisomy 16 and human trisomy 21 are not totally identical, the underlying molecular mechanisms of dysmorphogenesis induced by the trisomic state can be further investigated using the mouse model. Here the production of transgenic mice carrying only single genes or gene sequences from the mouse and human chromosome region will help elucidate which genes are responsible for the specific malformation pattern encountered in human and animal aneuploidies.

The relevance of this information becomes more evident if one takes into consideration that every year thousands of trisomy 21 pregnancies are terminated. The number of pregnancy terminations due to chromosome imbalance has increased over the past 20 years because more patients seek genetic counseling and prenatal diagnosis. Thus, it is our responsibility to fully characterize the pathogenetic mechanisms of Down syndrome and to provide medical care to the affected patients rather than terminate trisomic pregnancies.

REFERENCES

1. Epstein CJ. *The Consequences of Chromosome Imbalance: Principles, Mechanisms and Models.* New York: Cambridge University Press; 1986.
2. Epstein CJ. The consequences of chromosome imbalance. *Am J Med Genet.* 1990;7(3):31–37.
3. Reeves RH, Gearhart JD, Littlefield JW. Genetic basis for a mouse model of Down syndrome. *Brain Res Bull.* 1986;16:803–814.
4. Cox DR, Epstein LB, Epstein CJ. Genes coding for sensitivity to interferon (IFRec) and soluble superoxide dismutase (SOD-1) are linked in mouse and man and map to mouse chromosome 16. *Proc Natl Acad Sci USA.* 1980;77:2168–2172.

5. Reeves RH, Gallahan D, O'Hara BF, Callahan R, Gearhart JD. Genetic mapping of Prm-1, Igl-1, Smst, Mtv-6, SOD-1, Ets-2 and localization of the Down syndrome region on mouse chromosome 16. *Cytogenet Cell Genet.* 1987;44:76–81.
6. Gardiner K, Watkins P, Münke M, Drabkin H, Jones C, Patterson D. Partial physical map of human chromosome 21. *Somat Cell Mol Genet.* 1988;14:623–638.
7. Horisberger MA, Wathelet M, Szpirer J, et al. cDNA cloning and assignment to chromosome 21 of IFI-78K gene, the human equivalent of murine Mx-gene. *Somat Cell Mol Genet.* 1988;14:123–131.
8. Warren AC, Slaugenhaupt SA, Lewis JG, Chakravarti A, Antonarakis SE. A genetic linkage map of 17 markers on human chromosome 21. *Genomics.* 1989;4:579–591.
9. Irving NG, Hardy JA, Brown SDM. The multipoint genetic mapping of mouse chromosome 16. *Genomics.* 1991;9:386–389.
10. Reeves RH, Crowley MR, Lorenzon N, Pavan WJ, Smeyne RJ, Goldowitz D. The mouse neurologic mutant weaver maps within the region of chromosome 16 that is homologous to human chromosome 21. *Genomics.* 1989;5:522–526.
11. Moisan JP, Mattei MG, Mandel JL. Chromosome localization and polymorphism of an oestrogen-inducible gene specifically expressed in some breast cancers. *Hum Genet.* 1988;79:168–171.
12. Münke M, Kraus JP, Ohura T, Francke U. The gene for cystathionine b-synthetase (CBS) maps to the subtelomeric region on human chromosome 21q and to proximal mouse chromosome 17. *Am J Hum Genet.* 1988;42:550–559.
13. Burmeister M, Kim S, Proce ER, Lange T de, Tantravahi U, Myers RM, Cox DR. A map of the distal region of the long arm of human chromosome 21 constructed by radiation hybrid mapping and pulse-field gel electrophoresis. *Genomics.* 1991;9:19–30.
14. Threadgill DS, Kraus JP, Krawetz SA, Womack JE. Evidence for the evolutionary origin of human chromosome 21 from comparative mapping in the cow and mouse. *Proc Natl Acad Sci USA.* 1991;88:154–158.
15. Holtzman DM, Bayney RM, Li Y, Khosrovi H, Berger CN, Epstein CJ, Mobley WC. Dysregulation of gene expression in mouse trisomy 16, an animal model of Down syndrome. *EMBO.* 1992;11(2):619–627.
16. Bacchus C, Sterz H, Buselmaier W, Sahai S, Winking H. Genesis and systematization of cardiovascular anomalies and analysis of skeletal malformations in murine trisomy 16 and 19. Two animal models for human trisomies. *Hum Genet.* 1987;77:12–22.
17. Sterz H, Buselmaier W, Bacchus C, Gromier L, Eppler E. Defects of skeletal morphology, density and structure in mouse fetuses with trisomy 16. *Teratology.* 1989;40:627–639.
18. Miyabara S. Cardiovascular malformations of mouse trisomy 16: pathogenetic evaluation as an animal model for human trisomy 21. In: Clark EB, Takao A, eds. *Developmental Cardiology: Morphogenesis and Function.* Mt. Kisco, NY: Futura Publishing; 1990:409–430.
19. Buselmaier W, Bacchus C, Sterz H. Genesis and systematization of cardiovascular anomalies in murine trisomy 16. In: *The Morphogenesis of Down Syndrome.* New York: Wiley-Liss; 1991:203–214.

20. Gropp. A, Kolbus U, Giers D. Systematic approach to the study of trisomy in the mouse II. *Cytogenet Cell Genet.* 1975;14:42–62.
21. Binder M. The teratogenic effects of a bis (dichloroacetyl) diamine on hamster embryos: aortic arch anomalies and the pathogenesis of the DiGeorge syndrome. *Am J Pathol.* 1985;118:179–193.
22. Hackensellner HA. Arteria subclavia lusoria bei einem 14.5 mm langen menschlichen Embryo. *Anat Anz.* 1955;102:204–209.
23. Okamoto N. Cardiac morphogenesis and teratogenesis. *Congen Anom.* 1988;28:S103–S117.
24. Kirby ML, Bockman DE. Neural crest and normal development: a new perspective. *Anat Rec.* 1984;209:1–6.
25. Van Mierop LHS, Kutsche LM. Cardiovascular anomalies in DiGeorge syndrome and importance of the neural crest as a possible pathogenetic factor. *Am J Cardiol.* 1986;58:133–137.
26. Rugh R. *The Mouse: Its Reproduction and Development.* Minneapolis: Burgess; 1968.
27. Van Mierop LHS. Embryology of the atrioventricular canal region and pathogenesis of endocardial cushion defects. In: Feldt RH, ed. *Atrioventricular Canal Defect.* Philadelphia: WB Saunders; 1976:1–12.
28. Pexieder T, Miyabara S, Gropp A. Congenital heart disease in experimental (fetal) mouse trisomies: incidence. In: Pexieder T, ed. *Perspectives in Cardiovascular Research.* New York: Raven Press; 1981:5: 389–399.
29. Warkany J, Passarge E, Smith LB. Congenital malformations in autosomal trisomy syndromes. *Am J Dis Child.* 1966;112:502–517.

—————————— Chapter 7 ——————————

THE HEART IN
DOWN SYNDROME
Pathologic Anatomy

Richard Van Praagh, John Papagiannis,
Yaron I. Bar-El, and Oscar A. Schwint

B ASED ON THE CLASSICAL STUDY of Rowe and Uchida (1), it has long been assumed 1) that congenital heart disease occurs in approximately 40% of individuals with Down syndrome; and 2) that of those with congenital heart disease, common atrioventricular canal and ventricular septal defect are approximately equal in prevalence.

However, in a population-based study referred to by Greenwood and Nadas (2), a much higher prevalence of congenital heart disease was found in individuals with Down syndrome (62.3%). Moreover, these workers observed that common atrioventricular canal was much more frequent than isolated ventricular septal defect. In 230 patients with Down syndrome and congenital heart disease studied at Children's Hospital in Boston from 1962 to 1973, common atrioventricular canal was found in 48.7%, whereas isolated ventricular septal defect occurred in only 28.7% (2). In the population-based study of the New England Regional Infant Cardiac Program—based on the six New England states of the United States from 1968 to 1973—an even more striking predominance of common atrioventricular canal was found: Common atrioventricular canal was noted in 56.5% and isolated ventricular septal defect in only 17.1% (2).

The main purpose of the present study was to attempt to delineate with clarity the various anatomic types of congenital heart disease that are associated with Down syndrome. We also sought to ascertain the relative prevalences of these various forms of congenital heart disease and to assess whether the findings of our hospital-based study are similar to or significantly different from those of population-based studies. Finally, we sought to establish whether there are any significant differences between common atrioventricular canal in patients with Down syndrome and in individuals without Down syndrome.

The records of 100 postmortem cases of Down syndrome with congenital heart disease were reviewed and the autopsied heart specimens of 89 of these 100 cases, retained in the Cardiac Registry of the Children's Hospital in Boston, were available for reexamination. In order to make these 100 cases as unselected as possible, they were chosen at random alphabetically. These 100 postmortem examinations were performed over a 43-year period from 1949 to 1991 inclusive. The sex of one patient was unknown. Of the remaining 99 patients, 40 (40.4%) were male and 59 (59.6%) were female, so that the male/female ratio was 40/59 (0.7). The median age at death was 7 months, the mean age was 3.7 years, and the range was from 19 weeks' gestation (youngest aborted fetus) to 41 years of age. The age at death was unknown in two of these 100 cases.

In order to compare common atrioventricular canal in patients with and without Down syndrome, a comparative study was performed based on 115 randomly selected postmortem heart specimens of patients having common atrioventricular canal but without Down syndrome.

Nonparametric analysis using the χ^2 criterion with the Yates correction was employed, a p value $< .05$ being regarded as statistically significant. Fisher's exact test was used when appropriate. A parametric method of analysis such as Student's t test was not used because we do not know that the populations, from which our patients with and without Down syndrome came, were normally distributed.

CLASSIFICATION AND TERMINOLOGY

Concerning common atrioventricular canal, the terminology and classification of Edwards (3), Bharati et al. (4), and Rastelli et al. (5) were used.

Complete Form

In the complete form of common atrioventricular canal, there is a ventricular septal defect of the atrioventricular canal type that is confluent with an ostium primum type of atrial septal defect, which together constitute an atrioventricular septal defect. The atrioventricular septal defect is the defect in the septum of the atrioventricular canal. The mitral and tricuspid valves are in common, that is, undivided.

In Type A complete common atrioventricular canal of Rastelli et al. (5), the anterosuperior leaflet of the common atrioventricular valve is divided and attached to the ventricular septal crest (Figure 1). In Type B complete common atrioventricular canal, the anterosuperior leaflet of the common atrioventricular valve is partly divided and is not attached to the crest of the muscular ventricular septum; instead it is attached via a papillary muscle to the right ventricular septal surface (Figure 2A) (5). In fact, in the infrequent Type B complete common atrioventricular canal, the anterior papillary muscle of the right ventricle may appear to arise from the right ventricular septal surface because the moderator band often is short or absent (Figure 2B). In Type C complete common atrioventricular canal, the anterosuperior bridging leaflet of the common atrioventricular valve is undivided and the free margin of this leaflet is unattached to the ventricular septal crest (Figure 3) (5).

Incomplete Forms

There are several incomplete forms of common atrioventricular canal. The most common is the ostium primum type of atrial septal defect with a cleft mitral valve (Figure 4). The superior and inferior leaflets of the valve of the atrioventricular canal have fused with each other, resulting in separate tricuspid and mitral annuli, and there is no ventricular septal defect of the atrioventricular canal type beneath the septal leaflet of the tricuspid valve (Figure 4A). From the left ventricular aspect (Figure 4B), the cleft (or, if wide, the gap) between the superior and inferior components of what normally is the anterior mitral leaflet is well seen.

Other less frequent forms of incomplete common atrioventricular canal include the following:

1. An isolated primum type of atrial septal defect, typically small, without a cleft anterior leaflet of the mitral valve
2. An isolated cleft of the anterior mitral leaflet, the cleft being of the common atrioventricular canal type, but without a primum type of atrial septal defect and without a ventricular septal defect of the atrioventricular canal type
3. An isolated ventricular septal defect of the atrioventricular canal type, without a cleft mitral valve and without an ostium primum type of atrial septal defect (with or without hypoplasia of the

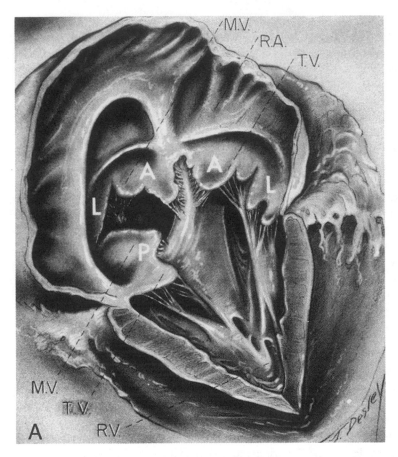

Figure 1. **A:** Type A complete common atrioventricular canal, right atrial (RA) view. The anterior leaflet of the common atrioventricular valve is divided into two components (A and A). The divided anterior leaflet (A, A) is attached to the crest of the muscular ventricular septum via numerous short chordae tendineae. The posterior leaflet (P) of the common atrioventricular valve is also attached to the crest of the ventricular septum via numerous short chordae. Despite the chordal attachments, a ventricular septal defect of the atrioventricular canal type exists through the thicket of chordae tendineae. The components of the tricuspid valve (TV) and of the mitral valve (MV) are readily recognizable, despite the fact that the atrioventricular valve is in common (unfused). In addition to the anterior (A) and posterior (P) leaflets of the common atrioventricular valve, there are also left lateral (L) and right lateral (R) leaflets. The potential TV opens into the morphologically right ventricle (RV) and the potential MV opens into the left ventricle (largely unseen). The septal band of the right ventricular septal surface (unlabeled) is shown prominently, whereas the ventricular sinus septum, posteroinferior to the septal band, is in shadow. (This photograph is reprinted by permission of [5] Rastelli GC, Kirklin JW, Titus JL. Anatomic observations on complete form of persistent common atrioventricular canal with special reference to atrioventricular valves. *Mayo Clin Proc.* 1966;41:296–308.)

Figure 1. (*continued*)

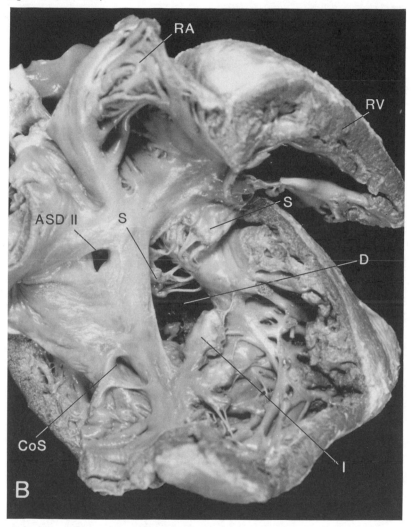

Figure 1. **B:** Type A complete common atrioventricular canal (CCAVC), showing opened RA and RV. The superior (anterior) leaflet (S) of the common atrioventricular valve (CAVV) is divided (S and S) and attached to the ventricular septal crest. The inferior (posterior) leaflet (P) also is well seen. The atrioventricular septal defect (D) (i.e., the defective septum of the atrioventricular canal) consists of an ostium primum type of atrial septal defect (between the atrial septum posterosuperiorly and the leaflets of the CAVV anteroinferiorly) and of a ventricular septal defect (VSD) of the atrioventricular canal (AVC) type (between the leaflets of the CAVV and the crest of the muscular ventricular septum). Note the spaces between the chordae tendineae of the leftward component of the superior leaflet (just in front of leftward S).

Figure 1. (*continued*)

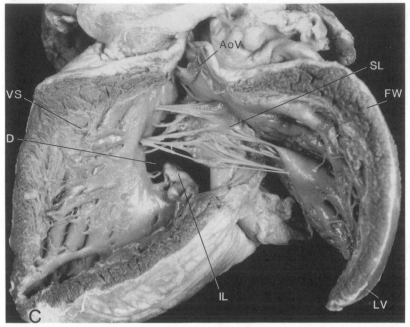

Figure 1. **C:** Type A CCAVC, viewed from the opened morphologically left ventricle (LV). The superior leaflet (SL) component of what should have composed the superior portion of the anterior mitral leaflet attaches via multiple chordae tendineae into the crest of the muscular ventricular septum (VS). The inferior leaflet (IL) component of what should have been the inferior portion of the anterior mitral leaflet also attaches via multiple chordae to the crest of the VS. The interchordal spaces are patent, constituting a VSD anteroinferior to the superior and inferior leaflet components. AoV, aortic valve; D, atrioventricular septal defect; and FW, free wall. Note that there is direct fibrous continuity between the AoV and the SL of the CAVV.

right ventricular sinus, and with or without straddling tricuspid valve)

4. A transitional form of common atrioventricular canal (of Edwards [3]) is very similar to a typical primum type of atrial septal defect with a cleft mitral valve, except that there are a few very small ventricular septal defects of the atrioventricular canal-type—interstices between the chordae tendineae that attach densely to the ventricular septal crest

5. The intermediate type of common atrioventricular canal (of Lev et al. [4]), in which the superior and inferior leaflets are fused in the midline (hence the common atrioventricular canal is not completely in common) but in which there typically is a large primum type of atrial septal defect and a large ventricular septal defect of the atrioventricular canal type

Figure 1. (*continued*)

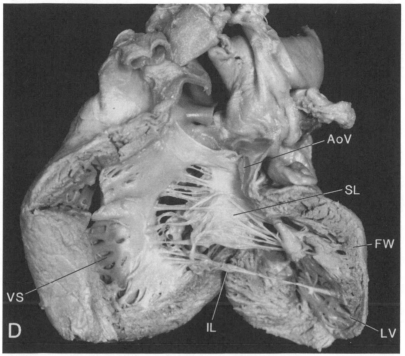

Figure 1. **D:** Type A CCAVC, LV view, showing multiple attachments of SL component and IL component of CAVV to crest of muscular VS. Other abbreviations as previously.

6. An Ebstein-like anomaly of the tricuspid valve, with or without tricuspid atresia, with no ventricular septal defect of the atrioventricular canal type, in association with a primum atrial septal defect and a cleft mitral valve opening into the left ventricle (encountered rarely)

The right-sided type of common atrioventricular canal (of Bharati et al. [4]) opens mostly into a large morphologically right ventricle and, to a much lesser degree, into a small morphologically left ventricle. The left-sided type of common atrioventricular canal (of Bharati et al. [4]) opens predominantly into a large morphologically left ventricle and, to a much lesser degree, into a small morphologically right ventricle. The right-sided and left-sided forms of common atrioventricular canal are often called unbalanced forms of common atrioventricular canal (of Bharati et al. [4]), as opposed to the *balanced form* of common atrioventricular canal that opens approximately equally into both the right and left ventricles.

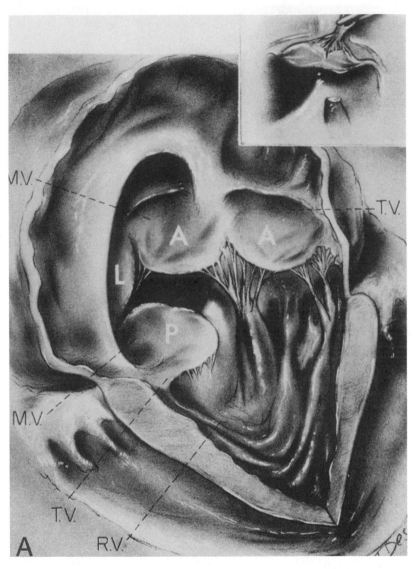

Figure 2. **A:** Type B complete common atrioventricular canal viewed from the right atrium. The anterior (superior) leaflet of the common atrioventricular valve is divided into two components (A and A). Neither component is attached to the crest of the muscular ventricular septum, as the inset shows. Instead the subdivided anterior leaflet (A, A) attaches via chordae tendineae to a right ventricular papillary muscle. The posterior (P) or inferior leaflet and the left lateral leaflet (L) of the common AV valve are also well seen. The unfused components of the mitral valve (MV) and tricuspid valve (TV) are readily appreciated. Normally, when the leftward A and the leftward part of P fuse, the composite anterior leaflet of the MV composed of A and P is formed. L becomes the posterior leaflet of the MV. The rightward portion of P normally becomes the septal leaflet of the TV, whereas the rightward A becomes the anterior leaflet of the TV. The posterior leaflet of the TV is not shown. (This photograph is reprinted by permission of [5] Rastelli GC, Kirklin JW, Titus JL. Anatomic observations on complete form of persistent common atrioventricular canal with special reference to atrioventricular valves. *Mayo Clin Proc.* 1966;41: 296–308.)

Figure 2. (*continued*)

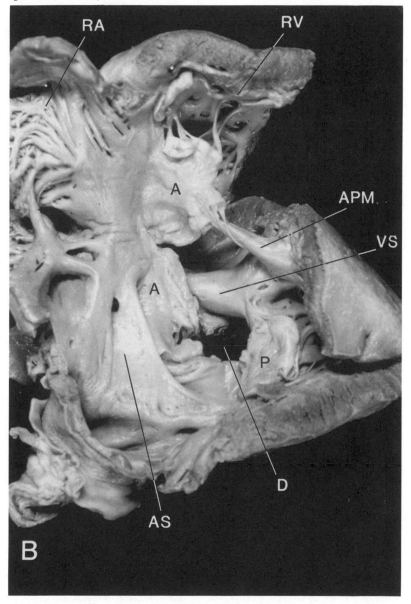

Figure 2. **B:** Case of the rare type B form of complete common atrioventricular canal (not encountered in these 100 randomly selected cases of Down syndrome and congenital heart disease). The anterior (superior) leaflet of the common atrioventricular valve is subdivided (A and A) but is not attached to the crest of the ventricular septum (VS). Instead, the subdivided anterosuperior leaflet is attached to the anterior papillary muscle (APM) of the right ventricle (RV). The APM appears to arise almost directly from the right ventricular septal surface because the moderator band is characteristically short. The atrioventricular septal defect (D) extends from the atrial septum (AS) dorsally to the VS ventrally. There is also a small secundum type of atrial septal defect (unlabeled, above the AS leader).

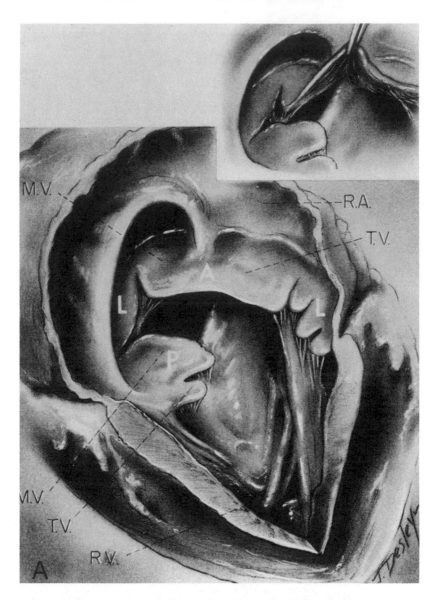

Figure 3. **A:** Type C complete common atrioventricular canal, right atrial view. The anterior leaflet (A) of the common AV valve is undivided and unattached to the crest of the muscular ventricular septum, as the inset confirms. The left and right lateral leaflets (L and L) and the posterior leaflet (P) of the common AV valve are also well seen. (This photograph is reprinted by permission of [5] Rastelli GC, Kirklin JW, Titus JL. Anatomic observations on complete form of persistent common atrioventricular canal with special reference to atrioventricular valves. *Mayo Clin Proc.* 1966;41:296–308.)

Figure 3. (*continued*)

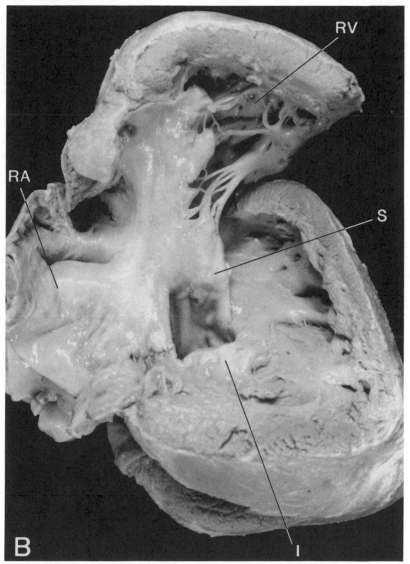

Figure 3. **B:** The opened right atrium (RA) and right ventricle (RV) showing that the superior leaflet (S) of the common AV valve is undivided. The inferior leaflet (I) is also easily seen. Note that the heart is shown in approximately the position that it would occupy in the chest in the sense that the diaphragmatic surface of the RV is parallel with the bottom of the photograph. The RA lies behind (not above) the RV. The RV apex points ventrally (not caudally). The superior leaflet (S) only becomes anterior if the heart is misoriented (i.e., if the ventricular apex is made to point at the patient's toes—which it does not in infants and children). Similarly, the inferior leaflet (I) only becomes posterior if the ventricular apex is made to point straight downward. Rotate the photograph 90° clockwise; only when misoriented in this way does the superior leaflet (S) become anterior relative to the inferior leaflet (I), which then becomes posterior. Note that in this conventional "apex-pointing-at-the-toes" misorientation, the diaphragmatic surface of the RV faces dorsally (the diaphragm would have to be vertical in this orientation!)—not caudally as it should. Accurately speaking, these leaflets are superior (not anterior) and inferior (not posterior). Nonetheless. in adolescents and adults, when the heart assumes a vertical or semivertical position (as opposed to the horizontal heart position of infancy and childhood), then the superior leaflet becomes anterior and the inferior leaflet becomes posterior.

Figure 3. (continued)

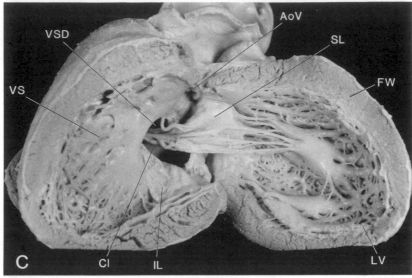

Figure 3. **C:** From the viewpoint of the opened left ventricle (LV), one can see that the superior leaflet (SL) is indeed undivided, that its *free margin* does not attach to the crest of the muscular ventricular septum (VS)—although one lone chorda does attach to the VS. The ventricular septal defect (VSD) part of the atrioventricular septal defect, not seen in B, is well seen. There is direct fibrous continuity between the aortic valve (AoV) and the SL of the common AV valve. The cleft (Cl) between the SL and the IL occupies an approximately horizontal plane, at right angles to the VS, which is typical of clefts of the AV canal type. By contrast, commissural clefts often point cephalically or vertically, not horizontally as canal clefts do.

FINDINGS

The 14 main cardiac diagnoses found in these 100 patients with Down syndrome and congenital heart disease who were studied postmortem are summarized in Table 1. It is noteworthy that Table 1 is a patient-based table that summarizes the main cardiac diagnosis in each of these 100 postmortem patients with Down syndrome and congenital heart disease. An anomaly-based table is presented in Table 3 on pages 98–99.

Common atrioventricular canal was by far the most frequent form of congenital heart disease associated with Down syndrome in this series: 63 cases (63%), Groups 1–4 inclusive (Table 1). The complete forms of common atrioventricular canal (52 cases, 52% of the series) were far more frequent than were the partial forms (11 cases, 11% of the series), the ratio of complete/partial forms being 4.7/1. Of the 52 cases of complete common atrioventricular canal, Type A (Figure 1) was present in 29 cases, Type B (Figure 2) in none, and Type C (Figure 3) in 23 cases.

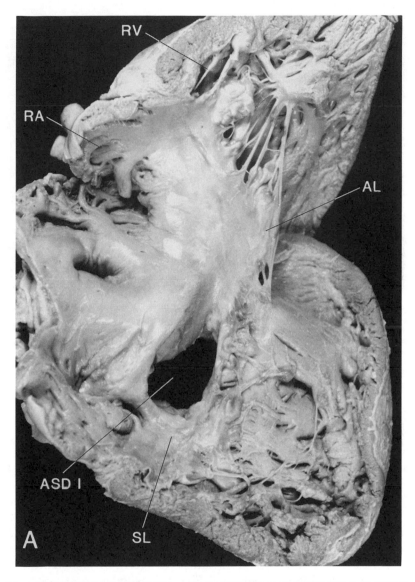

Figure 4.   Partial common AV canal (i.e., ostium primum type of atrial septal defect). **A:** Opened right atrial (RA) and right ventricular (RV) view of the classical partial form of common AV canal (i.e., ostium primum type of atrial septal defect [ASD I]). Note that there is no ventricular septal defect of the AV canal type beneath the septal leaflet (SL) of the tricuspid valve. The anterior leaflet (AL) of the tricuspid valve and the SL are fused—in direct fibrous continuity.

(continued)

Figure 4.   (continued)

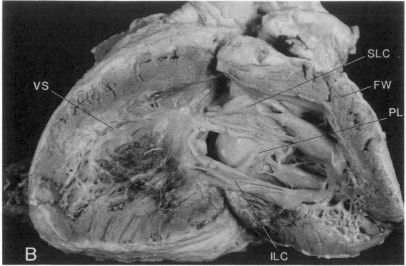

B

Figure 4.   **B:** The opened left ventricular (LV) view in another case of partial common AV canal of the ASD I type. There is a relatively large gap (not a cleft) between the superior leaflet component (SLC) and the inferior leaflet component (ILC) of the unfused anterior mitral leaflet, which resulted in severe mitral regurgitation. The posterior leaflet (PL) of the mitral valve is also well seen.

Of the 11 cases of partial common atrioventricular canal, ostium primum type of atrial septal defect with a cleft mitral valve (Figure 4) was present in six cases. The intermediate type (4) of common atrioventricular canal (with a primum type of atrial septal defect and a ventricular septal defect of the atrioventricular canal type, but with fusion of the superior and inferior leaflets of the atrioventricular canal in the midline) was found in one patient.

An isolated mitral valve cleft of the atrioventricular canal type (approximately at right angles to the left ventricular septal surface, as in Figure 5), without a primum type of atrial septal defect and without a ventricular septal defect of the atrioventricular canal type, was observed in three cases. A rare partial form of common atrioventricular canal was encountered (Figure 6) with an imperforate Ebstein type of anomaly resulting in tricuspid atresia (Figure 6B), a large secundum type of atrial septal defect (Figure 6C), a large primum type of atrial septal defect (Figure 6C), cleft mitral valve opening into the left ventricle (Figure 6D), no ventricular septal defect of the atrioventricular canal type (Figure 6D), a subaortic conoventricular type of ventricular septal defect (Figure 6D), and small-chambered right ventricle consisting mostly of a subpulmonary infundibulum (Figure 6A).

Table 1. The 14 main cardiac diagnoses in 100 postmortem cases of Down syndrome

Main anatomic diagnoses		Number of cases
1. Complete form of common AV canal		46
Type A	29	
Type B	0	
Type C	17	
2. Partial form of common AV canal		10
Ostium primum type of ASD	6	
Isolated mitral cleft	2	
Intermediate type	1	
Imperforate Ebstein	1	
3. Common AV canal and tetralogy of Fallot		7
Complete common AV canal	6	
Type A	0	
Type B	0	
Type C	6	
Partial common AV canal	1	
Cleft mitral valve	1	
4. Tetralogy of Fallot		8
5. Ventricular septal defect		12
6. Secundum atrial septal defect		9
7. Pulmonary atresia with intact ventricular septum		1
8. Pulmonary atresia with multiple small VSDs		1
9. Ebstein's anomaly		1
10. Tricuspid valve prolapse		1
11. Aortic valvar stenosis		1
12. Bicuspid aortic and pulmonary valves		1
13. Patent ductus arteriosus		1
14. Aberrant RSA and LSVC to CoS		1

Note: AV, atrioventricular; ASD, atrial septal defect; CoS, coronary sinus; LSVC, left superior vena cava; RSA, right subclavian artery; VSD, ventricular septal defects.

Percentages are omitted because number of cases = percentage of series.

It is noteworthy that one case of partial common atrioventricular canal occurred in the group of common atrioventricular canal with tetralogy of Fallot (Group 3). Hence, 10 cases of partial common atrioventricular canal occurred with normally related great arteries (Group 2), whereas one case of partial common atrioventricular canal was associated with tetralogy (Group 3).

In addition to complete common atrioventricular canal (the main cardiac diagnosis in 46 patients [see Table 1]) and partial common

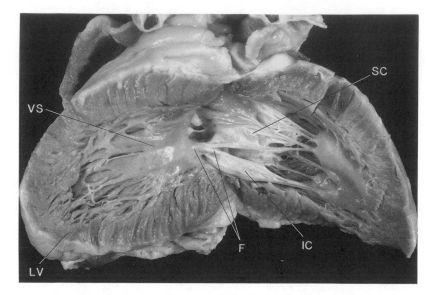

Figure 5. Partial cleft of anterior leaflet of mitral valve in a 35-year-old woman with Down syndrome and an ostium primum type of atrial septal defect (ASD I), opened left ventricular (LV) view. Note that paraseptally the superior component (SC) and inferior component (IC) of the anterior mitral leaflet are fused (F). The cleft is partial in the sense that it does not extend all the way from the free margin of the anterior mitral leaflet to the left ventricular septal surface (VS), as the cleft usually does in ASD I. The existence of partial clefts in the anterior leaflet of the mitral valve is part of the proof that the SC and the IC are parts of the anterior mitral leaflet (i.e., that the SC and the IC are not separate and independent leaflets in their own right). The anterior mitral leaflet (AML) is a composite structure. Normally, AML = SC + IC. In common AV canal, the fusion of SC and IC is partially or completely absent.

atrioventricular canal (the main cardiac diagnosis in 11 patients, 10 being isolated and one being associated with tetralogy of Fallot [Table 1]), what did the other 43 cases have? As is summarized in Table 1, common atrioventricular canal and tetralogy of Fallot coexisted in seven patients (one with isolated mitral cleft of the atrioventricular canal type mentioned above). Tetralogy of Fallot (isolated [i.e., without additional significant congenital heart disease]) occurred in eight cases. Ventricular septal defect (isolated) was found in only 12 patients. Secundum atrial septal defect was the only significant congenital heart disease in nine patients. Finally, one patient each had the following main cardiac diagnoses: pulmonary atresia with intact ventricular septum; pulmonary atresia with multiple small muscular and atrioventricular canal–type ventricular septal defects; Ebstein's anomaly; tricuspid valve prolapse; aortic valvar stenosis; bicuspid aortic and pulmonary valves; patent ductus arteriosus; and aberrant right subclavian artery with persistent left superior vena cava to coronary sinus.

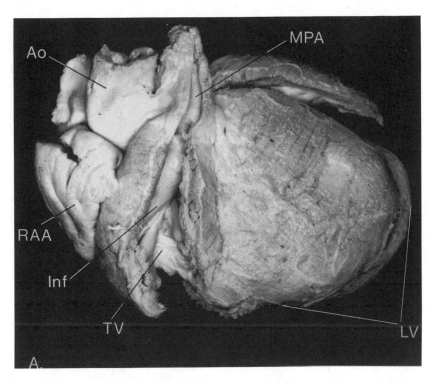

Figure 6. Partial common AV canal with imperforate Ebstein anomaly resulting in tricuspid atresia. **A:** Frontal view showing large left ventricle (LV) and underdeveloped right ventricle.

Each of the aforementioned groups is presented in greater detail in the following sections.

Complete Common Atrioventricular Canal

The malformations found in association with these 46 cases of complete common atrioventricular canal (Group 1, Table 1) are summarized in Table 2. The ratio of Type A:Type C complete common atrioventricular canal was 29:17 (1.7:1). Patent ductus arteriosus was the most common associated anomaly (18 cases, 39%), followed by secundum atrial septal defect (15 cases, 33%), persistent left superior vena cava to the coronary sinus (5 cases, 11%), double orifice of the potential mitral valve (4 cases, 9%), mitral regurgitation (4 cases, 9%), right-sided type of complete common atrioventricular canal (3 cases, 7%), preductal coarctation of the aorta (3 patients, 7% [see Table 2]), multiple congenital anomalies (2 cases, 4%), Hirschsprung disease (2 cases, 4%), and 14 other abnormalities in one case each.

Figure 6. (*continued*)

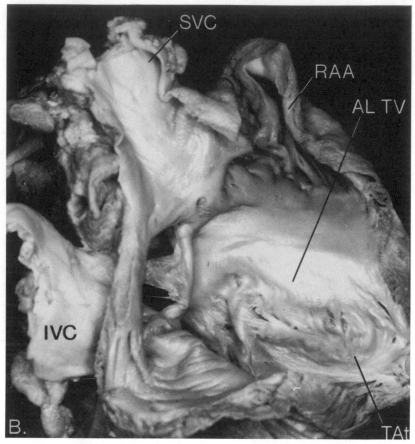

Figure 6. **B:** Right atrial view showing fusion of deep anterior leaflet of tricuspid valve (AL TV) with downwardly displaced septal leaflet resulting in tricuspid atresia (TAt). The small slit in the anterior tricuspid leaflet is a postmortem artifact.

Partial Common Atrioventricular Canal

The malformations associated with the 10 postmortem cases of Down syndrome with the partial form of common atrioventricular canal (Group 2) were as follows. A large mitral blood cyst was found in one patient with a primum type of atrial septal defect and a relatively huge gap (not a cleft) in the anterior mitral leaflet. The mitral gap was 10 mm wide at the left ventricular septal surface, where the blood cyst was also found within the unusually wide gap in this 14-month-old female. Large blood cysts of the leaflets were not found in complete common atrioventricular canal. In this patient, mitral regurgitation was severe. Mitral regurgitation was significant in 3 of

Figure 6. (*continued*)

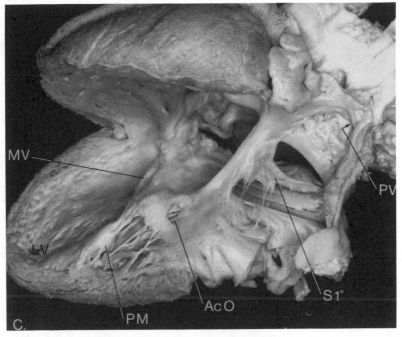

Figure 6. **C:** Left atrial and left ventricular view showing multiple large fenestrations of septum primum (S 1°) and a valve-incompetent foramen ovale, both of which constitute multiple large secundum atrial septal defects. A large ostium primum type of AV septal defect is confluent with the mitral valve (MV), which has a small accessory orifice (AcO) at the posteromedial commissure. Hence double-orifice mitral valve is present. PM, posteromedial papillary muscle; PV, pulmonary vein.

these 10 cases (30%), whereas mitral regurgitation was identified in only 9% of cases of complete common atrioventricular canal (Table 2). This is not a statistically significant difference ($p = .08$).

Incomplete mitral cleft was found in 3 of these 10 cases of the partial form of common atrioventricular canal (30%). The superior and inferior leaflet components were fused paraseptally (Figure 5). By definition, no case of incomplete cleft or partial fusion of the superior and inferior leaflet components was found in complete common atrioventricular canal. An aberrant right subclavian artery was found in 4 of these 10 cases of partial common atrioventricular canal (40%), whereas aberrant right subclavian artery occurred in only 2% of cases of complete common atrioventricular canal. This difference is statistically highly significant ($p = .003$). An Ebstein-like anomaly of the tricuspid valve occurred in two cases of partial common atrioventricular canal (20%), whereas an Ebstein-like anomaly was found

Figure 6. (continued)

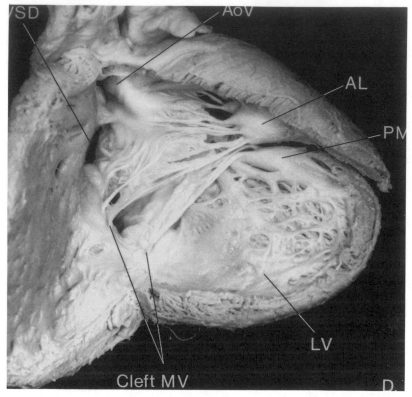

Figure 6. **D:** View of the opened LV and of the left ventricular outflow tract to the aortic valve (AoV). The cleft mitral valve (MV) is well seen, as is the "scooped out" configuration of the interventricular septum. A subaortic ventricular septal defect (VSD) is seen, this being a conoventricular type of VSD associated with anterior malalignment of the conal septum; no VSD of the AV canal type is present. Other abbreviations: Ao, aorta; AL, anterolateral papillary muscle of the left ventricle; Inf, infundibulum; IVC, inferior vena cava; PM, posteromedial papillary muscle of the left ventricle; RAA, right atrial appendage; and SVC, superior vena cava. (This photograph is reprinted with permission from the American College of Cardiology (*Journal of the American College of Cardiology,* 1991, 17, 932–943.)

in only 2% of the cases of complete common atrioventricular canal (Table 2). This difference is not statistically significant ($p = .07$). An imperforate Ebstein anomaly resulting functionally in tricuspid atresia occurred in one patient with a partial form of common atrioventricular canal (Figure 6). By definition, no form of tricuspid atresia occurred with complete common atrioventricular canal. Patent ductus arteriosus was somewhat less common in these cases of partial common atrioventricular canal (2 of 10 cases, 20%) than in complete

Table 2. Malformations associated with 46 cases of complete common atrioventricular canal in Down syndrome

Associated malformation	Number of cases	Percentage of series[a]
Type A	29	63
Type C	17	37
Patent ductus arteriosus	18	39
Secundum atrial septal defect	15	33
Left superior vena cava to CoS	5	11
Double-orifice mitral valve	4	9
Mitral regurgitation	4	9
Right-sided CCAVC	3	7
Preductal coarctation of the aorta	3	7
Multiple congenital anomalies	2	4
Hirschsprung aganglionic megacolon	2	4
Aortic fenestrations	1	2
Acute myelogenous leukemia	1	2
Aberrant right subclavian artery	1	2
Common atrium	1	2
DORV {S,D,D} with pulmonary conus	1	2
Ebstein-like anomaly of AL, RV	1	2
Familial Down syndrome	1	2
Left ventricular hypoplasia	1	2
LVOTO	1	2
Mitral stenosis	1	2
Single left ventricle, Holmes heart	1	2
Tracheal stricture, congenital	1	2
Translocation, 21–21	1	2
Tricuspid regurgitation	1	2

Note: AL, anterior leaflet; CCAVC, complete common atrioventricular canal; CoS, coronary sinus; DORV {S,D,D}, double-outlet right ventricle with segmental set of situs solitus of the viscera and atria, D-loop ventricles, and D malposition of the great arteries; LVOTO, left ventricular outflow tract obstruction (i.e., stenosis, not atresia).

[a]All percentages rounded off to the nearest whole number.

common atrioventricular canal (39%). This difference is not statistically significant ($p = .16$). Secundum atrial septal defect was found in 3 of these 10 cases of partial common atrioventricular canal (30%), a prevalence very similar to that in complete common atrioventricular canal (33%). Patent ductus arteriosus was present in two cases of partial common atrioventricular canal (20%) compared with 39% in complete common atrioventricular canal ($p = .16$, not a statistically significant difference).

In these 10 cases of partial common atrioventricular canal, there was one case each of the following: double-orifice mitral valve; left-sided type of common atrioventricular canal; multiple congenital anomalies; tricuspid regurgitation; and left ventricular hypoplasia.

Common Atrioventricular Canal and Tetralogy of Fallot

Common atrioventricular canal and tetralogy of Fallot coexisted in seven patients (7% of the series, Table 1) (Figure 7). In these seven patients, common atrioventricular canal was complete in six (86%) and partial in one (14%).

Interestingly, all seven patients had Rastelli Type C. One might object that the Rastelli classification (5) applies only to complete common atrioventricular canal and not to partial forms of common atrioventricular canal. We learned that this is not always so. In our one partial form of common atrioventricular canal with tetralogy (A52-198, a $15^{11}/_{12}$-year-old female), the anterosuperior leaflet of the atrioventricular valves was Type C: undivided, unattached to the ventricular septal crest, and continuous from mitral to tricuspid valve through a conoventricular type of ventricular septal defect. In other words, the ventricular septal defect was typical of tetralogy of Fallot—between the anterosuperiorly deviated conal septum above and the ventricular septum and septal band below, not a ventricular septal defect of the atrioventricular canal type. There was a complete cleft of the anterior leaflet of the mitral valve and very small primum

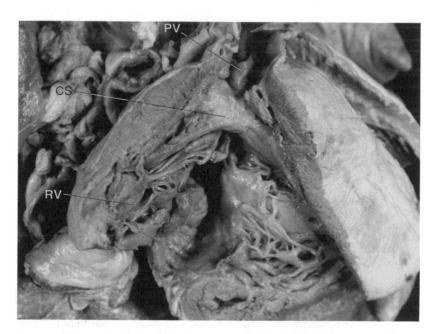

Figure 7. Complete common AV canal type C with tetralogy of Fallot. Note the anterior, superior, and leftward malalignment of the conal septum (CS), typical of tetralogy. The ventricular septal defect is of the confluent conoventricular (outlet) and AV canal (inlet) type (7). PV, pulmonary valve; RV, right ventricle.

type of atrial septal defect (5 × 4 mm). The tricuspid valve was also cleft, there being a wider than usual space between the anterior and septal leaflets of the tricuspid valve. Hence, this was a rare partial form of common atrioventricular canal.

Another case of complete common atrioventricular canal and tetralogy had a very small primum atrial septal defect (A78-47, 4½-month-old female). Hence, two of these cases of common atrioventricular canal and tetralogy of Fallot had a very small primum atrial septal defect (29%). A remarkably small primum type of atrial septal defect, with complete or partial common atrioventricular canal, was found only in association with tetralogy of Fallot.

All of these cases had pulmonary outflow tract stenosis, with none having pulmonary outflow tract atresia or absence of pulmonary valve leaflets. The pulmonary valve was bicuspid (bicommissural) in four cases (57%), unicuspid (unicommissural) in one (14%). A right aortic arch was present in two of these seven patients (29%). Two of these seven cases also had a persistent left superior vena cava to the coronary sinus, a secundum atrial septal defect, and an aberrant right subclavian artery.

There was one case each of the following: "mitral" regurgitation; "tricuspid" regurgitation; conoventricular type of ventricular septal defect; premature closure of the ductus arteriosus (in a 23-week fetal abortus); patent ductus arteriosus; prematurity—a 24-day-old male (A82-81) with a birth weight of 680 g at 32 weeks' gestation; translocation (D/G); and multiple congenital anomalies (esophageal atresia, in the premature with D/G translocation). The latter patient (A82-81) also had coarctation of the aorta (i.e., definite isthmic hypoplasia)—a rare finding in association with tetralogy of Fallot, plus a small probe patent ductus arteriosus.

Tetralogy of Fallot

A total of 15 patients had tetralogy of Fallot. Eight patients (8%) had "isolated" tetralogy of Fallot (i.e., without complete or partial common atrioventricular canal) without other major cardiovascular malformation. Of these 15 patients, seven (47%) had common atrioventricular canal, as above, and eight (53%) did not. It is with the latter group of "isolated" tetralogy that we are now concerned.

Again, all patients had pulmonary outflow tract stenosis (not atresia), four having a bicuspid pulmonary valve and one a unicuspid pulmonary valve. Hence, of these 15 patients with tetralogy, a bicuspid (bicommissural) pulmonary valve was present in eight (53%) and a unicuspid (unicommissural) pulmonary valve in two (13%). The number of pulmonary commissures and hence valve leaflets was not determined with certainty in the other five patients. (Postoperatively, it can be difficult to determine with certainty the number of commissures that were present preoperatively.)

A secundum type of atrial septal defect (i.e., pentalogy of Fallot) was found in three of these eight patients (37.5%). Hence, in these 15 patients with tetralogy as a whole (with and without common atrioventricular canal), a secundum type of atrial septal defect was present in five (33%). Thus, the prevalence of secundum atrial septal defect in tetralogy of Fallot seems not to be influenced by the presence or absence of common atrioventricular canal. It will be recalled that the prevalence of secundum atrial septal defect in complete plus partial common atrioventricular canal (Groups 1 and 2, Table 1) was 32%. Hence, in Down syndrome with common atrioventricular canal and/or tetralogy, about one third of these patients also had a secundum atrial septal defect.

A right aortic arch was found in two of these eight patients (25%). Among these 15 patients with tetralogy of Fallot as a whole, a right aortic arch was present in four (27%). A right aortic arch was found only in association with tetralogy of Fallot.

In these eight patients with "isolated" tetralogy, there was one patient each with the following: aberrant right subclavian artery (with left aortic arch); aberrant left subclavian artery (with right aortic arch); left superior vena cava to coronary sinus; multiple congenital anomalies (annular pancreas); familial Down syndrome (also present in the patient's paternal cousin); aortic regurgitation due to marked underdevelopment of the right coronary-noncoronary commissure, resulting in a bicuspid (bicommissural) aortic valve with one long and redundant leaflet (right coronary and noncoronary leaflets in undivided continuity) and one short and higher leaflet (left coronary); absent ductus arteriosus; high left coronary ostium; obstructed ventricular septal defect produced by redundant tricuspid leaflet tissue, resulting in a suprasystemic right ventricle (i.e., right ventricular systolic pressure higher than systemic pressure); seizure disorder; and vascular ring (right aortic arch with left ligamentum arteriosum).

Ventricular Septal Defect

"Isolated" ventricular septal defect (i.e., without tetralogy of Fallot and without common atrioventricular canal) occurred in 12 patients with Down syndrome (12%, Group 5 in Table 1). Of these 12 patients, a ventricular septal defect of the conoventricular type (between the conal septum above and septal band below) occurred in 11, and a small muscular ventricular septal defect (1 mm in diameter) occurred in one, a 36-hour-old female who was the infant of a diabetic mother.

Of these 11 conoventricular type of ventricular septal defects, conal septal hypoplasia of mild to moderate degree was found in 7 of 11 patients (64%). Mild anterior malalignment of the conal septum was also present in 3 of 11 patients (27%). The ventricular septal defect was purely membranous in 2 of 11 patients (18%) (i.e., the conal septum appeared entirely normal without any hypoplasia or malalignment), and consequently the ventricular septal defect appeared to be the result of an anomaly of the membranous septum, not the conal septum (hypoplasia ± malalignment), the latter being the usual situation. Hence, the purely membranous type of conoventricular septal defect was notably infrequent.

An aneurysm of the membranous septum was found in 2 of 11 patients with conoventricular septal defect. The membranous portion of the interventricular septum appeared to be produced by the superior leaflet of the common atrioventricular valve, just above its point of fusion with the inferior leaflet. Hence, the membranous septum appeared to consist of superior atrioventricular cushion leaflet tissue between the anterior and septal tricuspid leaflets. When prominent, this superior cushion paraseptal leaflet tissue formed a membranous septal aneurysm, which also constituted a prominent "infundibular" leaflet of the tricuspid valve anterosuperiorly (i.e., between the anterior and the septal tricuspid leaflets).

A secundum type of atrial septal defect was found in 3 of these 12 patients (25%). The following anomalies occurred in 2 of these 12 patients (17%): persistent left superior vena cava to coronary sinus; patent ductus arteriosus; and aberrant right subclavian artery. Finally, one patient (8% of this group) had multiple congenital anomalies (duodenal atresia); familial Down syndrome (in a male twin of our patient, a $1^{3}/_{12}$-year-old boy, A73-5); and prematurity.

Secundum Atrial Septal Defect

There were nine patients whose main cardiac diagnosis was a secundum type of atrial septal defect (9% of the series). The sinus venosus type of atrial septal defect was not encountered in this series. Septum primum (the flap valve of the foramen ovale) was very deficient in six of nine cases (67%).

Other salient findings were patent ductus arteriosus in five patients (56%); a large but intact membranous septum in three (33%); and a persistent left superior vena cava to coronary sinus in two (22%). There was one patient each with the following (11% of atrial septal defect group): myxomatous and redundant tricuspid and mitral valve leaflets; nondysjunctional mosaic; aberrant right subclavian artery; multiple congenital anomalies (duodenal atresia); Meckel's diverticulum; prematurity; and premature closure of the ductus arteriosus by thrombus in a 19-week-old fetus.

Pulmonary Atresia with Intact Ventricular Septum

In this series of 100 postmortem cases of Down syndrome with congenital heart disease, one patient had pulmonary atresia with intact ventricular septum (1% of the series, Table 1). The patient was a 24-day-old female (A91-94) in whom Down syndrome was proved by karyotype. This patient also had double-orifice tricuspid valve with an accessory posterior orifice (measuring 3 mm in diameter, the main orifice measuring 12 mm in diameter), multiple (three) secundum atrial septal defects, and a patent ductus arteriosus. Because of marked tricuspid regurgitation, the right ventricle was of good size and there was no right ventricular endocardial fibroelastosis, no sinusoids, and no coronary arteriopathy. There were advanced maternal age and parity, the mother being a 43-year-old gravida 7 para 5.

Pulmonary Atresia with
Multiple Small Ventricular Septal Defects

A 27-day-old boy (A75-66) was found to have pulmonary atresia (valvar) with multiple very small ventricular septal defects. Two tiny muscular ventricular septal defects were located halfway between the ventricular apex and the base, at the junction of the ventricular septum with the anterosuperior ventricular free walls (just beneath the anterior descending coronary artery). In addition, there was a tiny slit-like ventricular septal defect of the atrioventricular canal type—so small as to be thought minimally patent from the functional standpoint. The tricuspid valve had an Ebstein-like deformity with mild to moderate downward displacement of the septal leaflet, a relatively deep anterior leaflet, and marked tricuspid regurgitation (Figure 8). In addition, there was a giant right atrium, common atrium, and a probe patent ductus arteriosus.

Ebstein's Anomaly

The main cardiac diagnosis was Ebstein's anomaly in one patient, a 1-week-old female (A71-174). This patient had Ebstein's anomaly with tricuspid stenosis (4 × 4 mm in internal diameter), which was associated with pulmonary valvar stenosis (bicuspid pulmonary valve), a small (3 × 3 mm) subaortic conoventricular type of ventricular septal defect, a secundum type of atrial septal defect due to

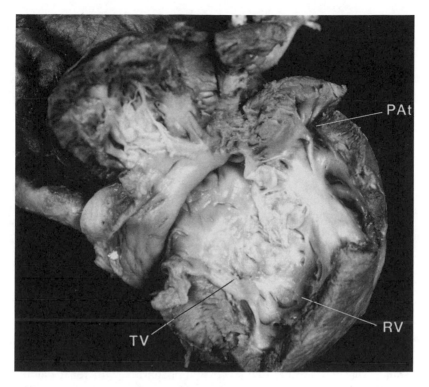

Figure 8. Pulmonary atresia (PAt) with dysplastic Ebstein-like tricuspid valve (TV) and multiple very small ventricular septal defects. The two small muscular VSDs and one slit-like VSD of the AV canal type were so small that the ventricular septum was thought to be functionally essentially intact. This is a rare form of congenital heart disease to be associated with Down syndrome (karyotype proved).

fenestrations in septum primum, absence of the ductus arteriosus, and a persistent left superior vena cava to the coronary sinus.

Tricuspid Valve Prolapse

One patient, a 9¾-month-old African American female (A88-5), had a deep curtain-like anterior leaflet of the tricuspid valve, no downward displacement of the septal leaflet, and marked redundancy and prolapse of the tricuspid valve leaflets—particularly of the anterior leaflet—resulting in severe tricuspid regurgitation. The mitral valve was also somewhat dysplastic; hence polyvalvular disease was present. Nonetheless it was the congenital tricuspid valve prolapse that was predominant. In addition, there was a large secundum atrial septal defect and a small patent ductus arteriosus. Terminal events were severe respiratory syncitial virus pneumonia and bradycardia with heart block that appeared 4 days prior to death.

Aortic Valvar Stenosis

The main cardiac diagnosis in one patient, a 5-week-old boy (A61-109), was congenital aortic valvar stenosis (1% of the series, Table 1). Stenosis was severe, there being only a 1- to 2-mm opening. The aortic valve was bicuspid (bicommissural) due to rudimentary development of the intercoronary commissure. The patient also had a secundum atrial septal defect.

Bicuspid Aortic and Pulmonary Valves

A 17$^7/_{12}$-year-old female (A65-266) with a D group to G group translocation had bicuspid semilunar valves bilaterally. The pulmonary valve had a rudimentary septal commissure (adjacent to the aortico-pulmonary septum) and the aortic valve had a rudimentary right coronary–noncoronary commissure. Bilaterally bicuspid semilunar valves is an unusual form of polyvalvular disease, and in this case it appeared not to be associated with any semilunar valvar dysfunction. Both semilunar valves also were fenestrated, but because the leaflet free margins were intact, significant semilunar regurgitation was thought not to have been present.

This young woman died of renal disease, not congenital heart disease. She had only one kidney, an ectopic presacral one that was thought probably to be the right kidney. The left ureter was a fibrous strand. She had chronic end-stage pyelonephritis with renal calcification, and she died of renal failure. Having a renal malformation, she had multiple congenital anomalies (i.e., malformations of more than one system—in this case the cardiovascular and the renal).

Patent Ductus Arteriosus

The main cardiac diagnosis in one patient, a 30-year-old woman (A66-107), was a large patent ductus arteriosus (8 mm in diameter). She also had a small conoventricular type of ventricular septal defect, a 1-mm opening in the membranous septum. This was not regarded as a purely membranous ventricular septal defect because the conal septum was also mildly hypoplastic. The conal septum should have been 36 mm in length (from the pulmonary valve above to the tricuspid valve below). Instead, the conal septum was only 27 mm long (from the pulmonary valve above to its inferior muscular rim above the tricuspid valve below). Hence, the inferior portion of the conal septum was foreshortened from 36 to 27 mm (a difference of 9 mm). Consequently, the degree of conal septal hypoplasia is 9/36 mm (25%). However, the large patent ductus was the predominant lesion. Autopsy revealed organizing pulmonary thrombi, right-sided bronchopneumonia, and a Meckel's diverticulum.

Aberrant Right Subclavian Artery and
Persistent Left Superior Vena Cava to the Coronary Sinus

One 12-day-old female (A51-34) had the above-mentioned anomalies as the main cardiac diagnosis. In addition, the patient had a very small secundum type of atrial septal defect. None of these cardiovascular abnormalities was thought to be clinically significant. This patient had duodenal atresia, which was the main clinical problem.

Cardiovascular Malformation-Based Analysis Table 3 is an anomaly-based (not a patient-based) summary of the findings in this study. The malformations are not ranked as primary (main) or secondary (associated) anomalies, as they are in Table 1. In Table 3, the findings are organized only in order of decreasing prevalence. We were surprised to find, for example, that secundum atrial septal defect was the second most common cardiovascular anomaly associated with Down syndrome (40%, Table 3). Table 3 provides information on the frequency of particular malformations, no matter whether the anomalies in question were regarded as main diagnoses or as associated findings.

Confidence intervals are included in an effort to answer the following question: How likely is it that the findings of the present study correspond to the true but unobserved proportions of these various anomalies in the population of individuals with Down syndrome who have congenital heart disease as a whole? A 95% confidence interval indicates that there is a 95% probability that the true but unobserved proportion of the anomaly in question lies within the specified interval.

Perhaps it should be added for clarity that conoventricular ventricular septal defects were found in 16 individuals (Table 3). This does not include patients with tetralogy of Fallot, who also have conoventricular defects with anterosuperior malalignment of the conal septum. For clarity, tetralogy of Fallot is presented separately (Table 3).

Common Atrioventricular Canal in Down Syndrome and in Patients Without Syndrome Because common atrioventricular canal was by far the most prevalent form of congenital heart disease in these 100 postmortem cases of Down syndrome (63%), we considered it worthwhile to compare and contrast Down syndrome versus non–Down syndrome common atrioventricular canal. Consequently, the 63 postmortem cases with Down syndrome common atrioventricular canal were compared with 115 postmortem cases of non–Down syndrome common atrioventricular canal, both groups being selected at random (Table 4). Four statistically highly significant differences were found (Table 4):

Table 3. Prevalence of various anomalies in series of 100 postmortem cases of Down syndrome with congenital heart disease

Anomaly	No. of cases (% of series)	Confidence interval (%)[a]
Complete common atrioventricular canal	52	42–62
Secundum atrial septal defect	40	30–50
Patent ductus arteriosus	35	26–44
Type A CCAVC	29	20–38
Type C CCAVC	23	15–31
VSD, conoventricular type	16	9–23
Left superior vena cava to coronary sinus	13	6–20
Aberrant right subclavian artery	12	6–18
Partial common atrioventricular canal	11	5–17
Tetralogy of Fallot	8	3–13
Mitral regurgitation	8	3–13
Multiple congenital anomalies	8	3–13
CAVC and tetralogy of Fallot	7	2–12
Tricuspid regurgitation	6	1–11
Prematurity	6	1–11
Double-orifice mitral valve	5	1–9
Ebstein-like anomaly	5	1–9
Right aortic arch	4	0–8
Convulsive disorder	4	0–8
Premature closure or absence of ductus arteriosus	4	0–8
Preductal coarctation of aorta	4	0–8
Large membranous septum, intact	3	0–6*
Familial Down syndrome	3	0–6*
Aneurysm of membranous septum, with VSD	3	0–6*
Isolated mitral valve cleft (no AVSD)	3	0–6*
Small primum atrial septal defect	2	1–3**
VSD, muscular	2	1–3**
Hirschsprung disease	2	1–3**
Potentially parachute mitral valve	2	1–3**
Common atrium	2	1–3**
Duodenal atresia	2	1–3**
Meckel's diverticulum	2	1–3**
Double-orifice tricuspid valve	1	0–2+
Congenital tricuspid stenosis	1	0–2+
Congenital mitral stenosis	1	0–2+
DORV {S,D,D} with subpulmonary conus	1	0–2+
Acute myelogenous leukemia	1	0–2+
Congenital tracheal stricture	1	0–2+
Intermediate type of CAVC	1	0–2+
Partial CAVC with imperforate Ebstein's	1	0–2+

(continued)

Table 3. (continued)

Anomaly	No. of cases (% of series)	Confidence interval (%)[a]
Partial CAVC, left-sided type	1	0–2[+]
Incomplete cleft of anterior mitral leaflet	1	0–2[+]
Blood cyst in mitral cleft	1	0–2[+]
Aortic regurgitation	1	0–2[+]
High origin of left coronary ostium	1	0–2[+]
Tetralogy of Fallot with obstructive VSD	1	0–2[+]
Infant of diabetic mother	1	0–2[+]
Intestinal obstruction at sigmoid colon	1	0–2[+]
Mosaic, nondysjunction	1	0–2[+]
Pulmonary atresia with intact ventricular septum	1	0–2[+]
Pulmonary atresia with multiple tiny VSDs	1	0–2[+]
Heart block, spontaneous, acquired	1	0–2[+]
Aortic stenosis, valvar	1	0–2[+]
Bicuspid and fenestrated semilunar valves	1	0–2[+]
Aberrant left subclavian artery with right AA	1	0–2[+]

[a]The 95% confidence intervals have no symbol beside them and apply when $n\hat{p}$ (the number of the proportion) $\geq$ 4. When $n\hat{p}$ = 3, no greater than a 90% confidence interval can be used, indicated by one asterisk (*). When $n\hat{p}$ = 2, only a 70% confidence interval is appropriate, indicated by two asterisks (**). When $n\hat{p}$ = 1, only a 50% confidence interval is appropriate, denoted by a plus sign (+). Confidence intervals of less than 95% are regarded as statistically not significant. All percentages are rounded off to the nearest whole number.

Note: AA, aortic arch; AVSD, atrioventricular septal defect; CAVC, common atrioventricular canal; CCAVC, complete common atrioventricular canal; DORV, double-outlet right ventricle; VSD, ventricular septal defect.

1. Complete common atrioventricular canal was much more frequent in Down syndrome canals (83%) than in non–Down syndrome canals (45%) ($p < .001$).
2. Type C complete common atrioventricular canal was much more frequent in Down syndrome canals (44%) than in non–Down syndrome canals (17%) ($p < .005$).
3. Hypoplastic left ventricle was much less frequent with Down syndrome canals (8%) than with non–Down syndrome canals (19%) ($p < .01$).
4. Left ventricular outflow tract obstruction was far less common with Down syndrome common atrioventricular canal (6%) than with non–Down syndrome common atrioventricular canal (35%) ($p < .001$).

Discussion Perhaps the most important finding of this study is that common atrioventricular canal (complete and partial) was by far the most frequent form of congenital heart disease associated with Down syndrome (63%, Table 1), much more common than was "iso-

Table 4. Comparison of common atrioventricular canal in postmortem patients with Down syndrome[a] and in postmortem patients without Down syndrome[b]

	Down Common AV canal		Non–Down Common AV canal		χ^2	p
	No.	%	No.	%		
Complete CAVC	52	83	52	45	23.34	<.001
Partial CAVC	11	17	63	55		
Type A CCAVC	29	56	43	83	8.85	<.005
Type C CCAVC	23	44	9	17		
Hypoplastic LV	5	8	22	19	7.84	<.01
LVOTO	4	6	41	35	21.95	<.001

[a]$n = 63$.
[b]$n = 115$.
Note: CAVC, common atrioventricular canal; CCAVC, complete common atrioventricular canal; LV, left ventricle; LVOTO, left ventricular outflow tract obstruction.

lated" ventricular septal defect (12%), the ratio of common atrioventricular canal to ventricular septal defect being 5.25:1. Our findings are very different from those of some previous workers (1,8–12) but closely similar to those of others (2,13,14) (Table 5). The question therefore becomes whom to believe.

At first glance, the present study appears to have two serious limitations:

1. It is a postmortem-based study. Hence, one would expect the findings to be skewed toward "badness"—that is, toward common atrioventricular canal and away from isolated ventricular septal defect.

Table 5. Common atrioventricular canal versus ventricular septal defect: comparison of previous investigations with present study

Authors	Common AV canal (%)	Isolated VSD (%)
Rowe and Uchida (1)	36	33
Warkany et al. (6)	36	49
Cullum and Liebman (7)	24.5	32
Laursen (8)	15	49
Park et al. (9)	43	32
Katlic et al. (10)	46	27
Tandon and Edwards (11)	60	29
Greenwood and Nadas (2)	56.5	17
Ferencz et al. (12)	60	16
Present study	63	12

Note: AV, atrioventricular; VSD, ventricular septal defect.

2. It is a hospital-based study, not a population-based study. Thus, the present investigation is not necessarily representative of the findings in the population of Down syndrome patients with congenital heart disease as a whole.

However, comparison of the findings of this study with those of two large population-based investigations of living patients (2,14) revealed no statistically significant differences (Table 6). Indeed, our findings are almost identical to those of the previous large population-based studies (2,14) (Table 6), supporting the conclusion that common atrioventricular canal is by far the most frequent form of congenital heart disease associated with Down syndrome. The findings of the present study are summarized in Tables 1–4 and will not be reiterated here.

Prevalence of Congenital Heart Disease in Down Syndrome Rowe and Uchida (1) concluded that only about 40% of individuals with Down syndrome have congenital heart disease. However, the New England Regional Infant Cardiac Program data reported by Greenwood and Nadas (2) indicated that congenital heart disease was found in 62% of individuals with Down syndrome. Hence, congenital heart disease in Down syndrome may well be more common than is generally assumed.

Down Syndrome Versus Non–Down Syndrome Common Atrioventricular Canal Individuals with Down syndrome tended to have a more primitive or less developed state of the atrioventricular canal than individuals with non–Down syndrome (Table 4):

1. Complete common atrioventricular canal (total failure of septation of the atrioventricular canal—the most primitive or least developed stage in the septational process) was much more common in Down syndrome (83%) than in non–Down syndrome (45%) ($p < .001$).

Table 6. Comparison of the prevalences of common atrioventricular canal and isolated ventricular septal defect in population-based investigations and in the present study

Studies	CAVC (%)	VSD (%)	p
New England RICP (2)	61	17	
Baltimore-Washington IS (14)	60	16	NS[a]
Present study	63	12	

[a]No statistically significant difference was found between the finding of the present study and those of two large population-based studies (2,14).

Note: CAVC, common atrioventricular canal; IS, Infant Study; RICP, Regional Infant Cardiac Program; VSD, ventricular septal defect.

2. Type C complete common atrioventricular canal (the most primitive or least developed form of complete common atrioventricular canal in which the anterosuperior leaflet of the common atrioventricular valve is neither subdivided nor attached to the ventricular septal crest; Figure 3) was much more common in Down syndrome (44%) than in non–Down syndrome (17%) patients ($p < .005$). In Type A complete common atrioventricular canal (Figure 1), septation of the atrioventricular canal has clearly begun, the anterosuperior leaflet of the common atrioventricular valve being divided and attached to the ventricular septum. Although Type A complete common atrioventricular canal was more frequent than Type C both in patients with Down syndrome and without Down syndrome (Table 4), Type A was much more common in non–Down syndrome cases (83%) than in patients with Down syndrome (56%) ($p < .005$).

3. As the leaflets of the common atrioventricular valve become attached to the ventricular septum, the probabilities of left ventricular inflow tract and outflow tract obstruction increase. Parenthetically, it is important to remember that the mitral valve forms an integral part of the left ventricular inflow and outflow tracts. Consequently, the more undeveloped (Type C) stage is less prone to left ventricular inflow tract and outflow tract obstruction than are the more developed (Type A, or ostium primum type of atrial septal defect) stages. Hence, the frequency of hypoplasia of left ventricle was greater in patients without Down syndrome (19%) than in patients with Down syndrome (8%) ($p < .01$, Table 4).

4. Similarly, the frequency of left ventricular outflow tract obstruction was much greater in non–Down syndrome patients (35%) than in Down syndrome patients (6%) ($p < .001$).

All of the four above-mentioned differences between Down syndrome and non–Down syndrome common atrioventricular canal (Table 4) appear to be related to a greater tendency toward lack of development ("primitiveness") of the atrioventricular canal in Down syndrome patients than in non–Down syndrome cases. *Why* this is so—why Down syndrome patients tend to have a more "primitive" (less developed) atrioventricular canal than do non–Down syndrome patients—remains unknown. It is hoped that molecular genetics may be able to clarify this matter.

Our findings concerning the differences between Down syndrome and non–Down syndrome common atrioventricular canal (Table 4) confirm and amplify the observations of Marino and his colleagues that were published by De Biase et al. (15) (see Chapter 10).

ANATOMIC AND TERMINOLOGY CONSIDERATIONS

1. The designation *common atrioventricular canal* is preferred to *atrioventricular septal defect* as the name for the malformation as a whole because atrioventricular septal defect is only part of the anomaly. The concept of common atrioventricular canal includes both parts of the malformation: the septal part (i.e., the atrioventricular septal defect) and the leaflet part (i.e., the cleft mitral and tricuspid leaflets).

2. *The mitral cleft* is indeed a cleft, not a commissure (16), as partial clefts prove (Figure 5). In partial common atrioventricular canal of the typical ostium primum type, the anterior mitral leaflet really is cleft—that is, unfused (Figure 4) or incompletely fused (Figure 5). The left atrioventricular valve in this situation is not a trileaflet valve because the superior and inferior parts of the anterior mitral leaflet are leaflet components or parts, not complete and separate leaflets. Again, this point is proved by the well-documented existence of partial clefts of the anterior mitral leaflet (Figure 5).

3. *Fusion* of the superior and inferior endocardial cushions of the atrioventricular canal is a developmental fact that has been well documented in humans (Figure 9) and in other mammals (Figure 10) (17).

4. A *commissure* can occur only between two different leaflets, not within a leaflet (Figure 5).

5. The *papillary musculature* is noteworthy in this regard. At a true commissure, one papillary muscle group pulls two leaflets together—as at the anterolateral and posteromedial commissures of the mitral valve. At a cleft, two papillary muscle groups pull two leaflet components apart (Figures 4 and 5). The etymology of *commissure* is revealing: *cum,* with or together; *mittere,* to send [Latin]. Hence, the literal meaning of commissure is to send together. At a commissure of an atrioventricular valve, the tensor apparatus brings or sends the leaflets together; it does not pull them apart. At a mitral cleft, the tensor apparatus pulls the superior and inferior leaflet elements apart, this being one of the causes of mitral regurgitation in partial common atrioventricular canal (Figures 4 and 5). Hence, often it is unfortunate that a mitral cleft is indeed a cleft rather than a commissure.

6. Common atrioventricular canal is at least in part, an *endocardial cushion defect*. Research concerning cell surface adhesiveness and galactyltransferase is endeavoring to characterize the precise nature of the endocardial cushion defect at the cellular and molecular levels.

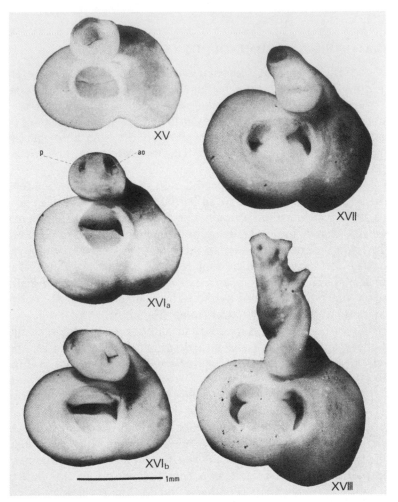

Figure 9.   Normal fusion of the common atrioventricular valve in humans. These dissected embryonic human hearts are viewed from above. The atria have been removed in order to make it possible to see the fusion of the superior and inferior endocardial cushions of the atrioventricular canal. The great arteries have been removed just above the semilunar valves, making it possible to see the normal morphogenetic movement of the semilunar valves. The Roman numerals indicate Streeter's horizons or developmental stages. The ventral surface of the heart faces the top of the page; the dorsal surface of the heart faces the bottom of the page; the right side of the heart corresponds to the viewer's right-hand side; and the left side of the heart corresponds to the viewer's left-hand side.

The superior (upper) and inferior (lower) endocardial cushions of the atrioventricular canal normally are not fused in horizon XV (30–32 days since ovulation) or in horizon XVI (32–34 days of age). Late in horizon XVI (XVIb, i.e., 33–34 days of age), one can see that the common atrioventricular valve opens predominantly into the left ventricle but also overrides the developing ventricular septum and opens a small amount into the developing right ventricle.

Normally, fusion of the superior and inferior endocardial cushions begins in horizon XVII (34–36 days of age). In horizon XVIII (36–38 days of age), one can see that the anterior mitral leaflet of this embryo remains partially cleft—adjacent to the free margin of the anterior mitral leaflet. In the malformation of common atrioventricular canal, this process of fusion either does not occur at all, resulting in completely common AV canal, or occurs only incompletely, resulting in partially common AV canal. Normally, the superior and inferior leaflets of the common AV valve fuse with each other (well seen here), and with the ventricular septum in front (not seen), and with the atrial septum behind (not seen). *Note:* ao, aortic valve; p, pulmonary valve. (This figure is reprinted by permission of [17] Asami I. Partitioning of the arterial end of the human heart. In: Van Praagh R, Takao A, eds. *Etiology and Morphogenesis of Congenital Heart Disease.* Mt Kisco, NY: Futura Publishing; 1980:51–61.)

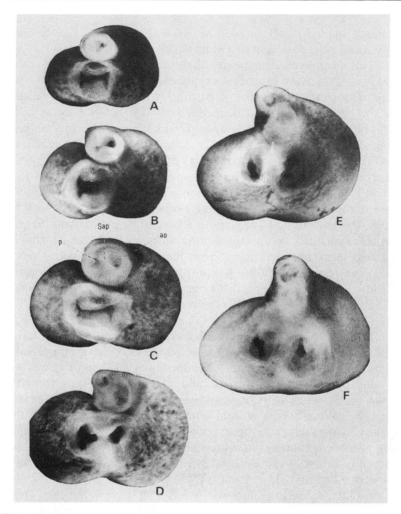

Figure 10. Normal fusion of the common atrioventricular valve in the rat. These embryonic rat hearts are dissected and viewed as in Figure 9. Again the fusion of the superior and inferior leaflets of the common AV valve is seen to contribute to the formation of a normally divided AV canal with separate mitral and tricuspid valves. **A:** 12-1/2 embryonic days of age; **B:** 12-3/4 days; **C:** 13 days; **D:** 13-3/4 days; **E:** 14-1/2 days; **F:** 15-1/2 days of age. Abbreviations as previously, except: Sap, septum aortopulmonale. (This figure is reprinted by permission of [17] Asami I. Partitioning of the arterial end of the human heart. In: Van Praagh R, Takao A, eds. *Etiology and Morphogenesis of Congenital Heart Disease*. Mt Kisco, NY: Futura Publishing; 1980: 51–61.)

DEVELOPMENTAL AND GENETIC CONSIDERATIONS

One of the more important developmental implications of the findings of the present study is that in order to understand the morphogenesis and the etiology of the congenital heart disease associated with Down syndrome, it may be necessary to understand the causation of many different cardiovascular anomalies (Tables 1 and 3), not just the embryology and the genetics of one or two malformations, such as common atrioventricular canal and ventricular septal defect.

This phenotypic complexity (Tables 1 and 3), however, could have a comparatively simple genotypic explanation. An attractive hypothesis, for example, is that of Kurnit—with whom the first author had the good fortune to work in the early 1980s—that *an increase in fibroblast cell surface adhesiveness* (18,19) explains the morphogenesis of common atrioventricular canal and ventricular septal defect. The idea is that as the fibroblasts of the endocardial cushions of the atrioventricular canal "take their random walks in space," as Kurnit put it, if there is an increase in the adhesiveness of the surface of these fibroblasts they will "like each other too much" and stick together, thereby failing to migrate to a normal degree. Subnormal migration results in a failure to form the atrioventricular canal septum, and also in a failure to zipper-close the cleft in the anterior mitral leaflet from medially (at the septum) to laterally (at the free margin of the anterior mitral leaflet). Computer modeling of this hypothesis of increased cell surface adhesiveness appeared to support this idea (18).

In order to test this hypothesis in tissue culture, the first author with the assistance of Matsuoka excised the developing mitral valve leaflet tissue from Down syndrome abortuses and this material was cultured. We were fascinated to find that the fibroblasts from the Down syndrome atrioventricular valve tissue did not migrate as well in tissue culture as did normal control fibroblasts. Reasoning that trisomy 21 typically was a total body abnormality, we then compared lung fibroblasts from Down syndrome abortuses with lung fibroblasts from non–Down syndrome normal controls. Again the findings were the same: The fibroblasts from the Down syndrome cases migrated subnormally in tissue culture, compared with normal controls. These tissue culture findings supported Kurnit's hypothesis of increased fibroblast cell surface adhesiveness, and they were published by Wright et al. in 1984 (19).

Lauer later told us that he and Runyan, a biochemist colleague, thought that this increase in cell surface stickiness may be mediated by galactyltransferase (often called "galtase").

Another important concept proposed by Kurnit et al. (20) is that cardiac morphogenesis may be influenced not only by genetics and resultant biochemistry but also by chance. This is known as the *stochastic (probabilistic) single-gene hypothesis,* as opposed to the multifactorial polygenic hypothesis. For example, in one of our cases of familial Down syndrome, a 1³/₁₂-year-old boy with Down syndrome and an Eisenmenger type of conoventricular ventricular septal defect

(A73-5) had a male twin with Down syndrome—but without congenital heart disease. Identical twins discordant for congenital heart disease, which is more the rule than the exception, clearly indicate that genes are not "everything" in the causation of congenital heart disease. Chance may play an important role (20).

But the burning question nonetheless remains: Where are the genes responsible for Down syndrome congenital heart disease? Korenberg and colleagues are doing exciting work in this regard (21). Korenberg thinks that a very small region at the distal end of the long arm of chromosome 21 is where the Down syndrome congenital heart genes are located, from q22.1 to q22.3 (21). Korenberg indicated that a very small region is involved, containing about 30 genes, only a subset of which is expressed in the embryonic heart (21).

Our present hope is that Korenberg and her colleagues will soon be able to identify and clone the gene or genes of Down syndrome congenital heart disease, aided by the recombinant DNA libraries created by Kurnit, using tissues dissected and obtained by the first author and Matsuoka. To our knowledge, this is essentially all that is known at the present time. This story is unfolding rapidly, but no one knows how it will end.

What patients with Down syndrome did not have may be, from the developmental standpoint, as important as what they did have:

1. We never found Down syndrome to be associated with situs inversus totalis.
2. Similarly, Down syndrome seems not to occur with situs ambiguus and the heterotaxy syndromes of congenital asplenia or polysplenia.
3. Down syndrome appears not to occur with segmental inversion (22). The cardiotype almost always is normal; that is, {S,D,S}, meaning the set of { } situs solitus of the viscera and atria {S,-,-}, D-loop or noninverted ventricles {-,D,-}, and solitus normally related great arteries {-,-,S} with a normal subpulmonary type of conus. Hence, the segmental set of the solitus normal heart is {S,D,S}, and this is what Down syndrome almost always has. Only one exception to the foregoing was encountered in this series, namely, a patient with double-outlet right ventricle {S,D,D}, denoting the set of situs solitus of the viscera and atria {S,-,-}, D-loop ventricles {-,D,-}, and D malposition of the great arteries {-,-,D}—that is, with a right-sided aortic valve. It was fascinating to see that even in this case (A75-29) there was a normal subpulmonary type of muscular conus, not the bilateral conus (subaortic and subpulmonary) that occurs so often with

double-outlet right ventricle. This 17-day-old boy also had a markedly hypoplastic left ventricle, aortic–common atrioventricular valvar direct fibrous continuity, and a Type C form of complete atrioventricular canal with the atrioventricular valve opening predominantly into the right ventricle (i.e., a right-sided type of common atrioventricular canal with a hypoplastic left ventricle). This is what Rowe and others (23) called infantile-type double-outlet right ventricle (because often the life expectancy is brief). This is due, at least in part, to the coexistence of a hypoplastic left heart. Had the left ventricle not been markedly hypoplastic, the appearance of double-outlet right ventricle might not have been present. Having a solitus normal type of conus, even this case of double-outlet right ventricle was not a genuine exception to the rule that *all of the cardiac segments in Down syndrome are in situs solitus.* Exceptions to this rule appear to be very rare; thus far we have not seen one.

4. We have never seen a case of typical transposition of the great arteries with a well-developed muscular subaortic conus and pulmonary-mitral fibrous continuity (22). Ferencz and colleagues (12) of the large Baltimore-Washington Infant Study agree. This we think is understandable because transposition typically has a very abnormal subaortic conus, whereas Down syndrome characteristically has a normal (subpulmonary) type of conus. The normal subpulmonary type of conus may be underdeveloped, resulting in tetralogy of Fallot (Table 1). However, the type of conus is basically normal (i.e., subpulmonary) even though it may be poorly expanded, as in tetralogy.

Hence, Down syndrome does not have "complex" congenital heart disease in the sense of multiple segmental situs mismatches. All of the cardiac segments were in situs solitus in the present study—even with tetralogy of Fallot and double-outlet right ventricle. Thus, Down syndrome congenital heart disease is very different from the heterotaxy syndromes (24) and very different from the *iv/iv* mouse model of situs inversus and situs ambiguus with polysplenia and occasionally with asplenia (25,26). The *iv* gene has recently been mapped to murine chromosome 12 (27,28), which corresponds to human chromosome 14.

In sharp contrast, Down syndrome seems to "guarantee" the presence of situs solitus of the viscera and of all cardiac segments. The *iv/iv* mouse model of the heterotaxy syndromes may functionally be regarded as a genetic "underdosage," a lack of genetic information with a loss of control of the development of normal laterality. Trisomy 21 may functionally be regarded as a genetic "overdosage" that guarantees situs solitus of the viscera and of all cardiac segments, but that may also cause a change in cell surface adhesive characteristics of fibroblasts, impeding their morphogenetic movements and interfering with their normal adhesion and fusion. The foregoing is our best current working hypothesis. It is understood that we still have much to learn.

REFERENCES

1. Rowe RD, Uchida IA. Cardiac malformation in mongolism, a prospective study in 184 mongoloid children. *Am J Med.* 1961;31:726–735.
2. Greenwood RD, Nadas AS. The clinical course of cardiac disease in Down's syndrome. *Pediatrics.* 1976;58:893–897.
3. Edwards JE. Congenital malformations of the heart and great vessels. A. Malformations of the atrial septal complex. In: Gould SE, ed. *Pathology of the Heart.* 2nd ed. Springfield, IL: Charles C Thomas; 1960: 260–293.
4. Bharati S, Lev M, McAllister HA, Kirklin JW. Surgical anatomy of the atrioventricular valve in the intermediate type of common atrioventricular orifice. *J Thorac Cardiovasc Surg.* 1980;79:884–889.
5. Rastelli GC, Kirklin JW, Titus JL. Anatomic observations on complete form of persistent common atrioventricular canal with special reference to atrioventricular valves. *Mayo Clin Proc.* 1966;41:296–308.
6. Van Praagh S, Vangi V, Sul JH, Metras D, Parness I, Castaneda AR, Van Praagh R. Tricuspid atresia or severe stenosis with partial common atrioventricular canal: anatomic data, clinical profile and surgical considerations. *J Am Coll Cardiol.* 1991;17:932–943.
7. Van Praagh R, Geva T, Kreutzer J. Ventricular septal defects: how shall we describe, name, and classify them? *J Am Coll Cardiol.* 1989;14: 1298–1299.
8. Warkany J, Passarge E, Smith LB. Congenital malformations in autosomal trisomy syndromes. *Am J Dis Child.* 1966;112:502–517.
9. Cullum L, Liebman J. The association of congenital heart disease with Down's syndrome (mongolism). *Am J Cardiol.* 1969;24:354–357.
10. Laursen HB. Congenital heart disease in Down's syndrome. *Br Heart J.* 1976;38:32–38.
11. Park SC, Mathews RA, Zuberbuhler JR, Rowe RD, Neches WH, Lenox CC. Down syndrome with congenital heart malformation. *Am J Dis Child.* 1977;131:29–33.
12. Katlic MR, Clark EB, Neill C, Haller JA. Surgical management of congenital heart disease in Down's syndrome. *J Thorac Cardiovasc Surg.* 1977;74:204–209.
13. Tandon R, Edwards JE. Cardiac malformations associated with Down's syndrome. *Circulation.* 1973;47:1349–1355.
14. Ferencz C, Neill CA, Boughman JA, Rubin JD, Brenner JI, Perry LW. Congenital cardiovascular malformations associated with chromosomal abnormalities: an epidemiologic study. *J Pediatr.* 1989;114:79–86.
15. De Biase L, DiCiommo V, Ballerini L, Bevilacqua M, Marcelletti C, Marino B. Prevalence of left-sided obstructive lesions in patients with

atrioventricular canal without Down's syndrome. *J Thorac Cardiovasc Surg.* 1986;91:467–472.

16. Anderson RH, Zuberbuhler JR, Penkoske PA, Neches WH. Of clefts, commissures, and things. *J Thorac Cardiovasc Surg.* 1985;90:605–610.
17. Asami I. Partitioning of the arterial end of the human heart. In: Van Praagh R, Takao A, eds. *Etiology and Morphogenesis of Congenital Heart Disease.* Mt Kisco, NY: Futura Publishing; 1980:51–61.
18. Kurnit DM, Aldridge JF, Matsuoka R, Matthysse S. Increased adhesiveness of trisomy 21 cells and atrioventricular canal malformations in Down syndrome: a stochastic model. *Am J Med Genet.* 1985;30: 385–399.
19. Wright TC, Orkin RW, Destrempes M, Kurnit DM. Increased adhesiveness of Down syndrome fetal fibroblasts in vitro. *Proc Natl Acad Sci USA.* 1984;81:2426–2430.
20. Kurnit DM, Layton WM, Matthysse S. Genetics, chance, and morphogenesis. *Am J Hum Genet.* 1987;41:979–995.
21. Korenberg JR, Bradley C, Disteche CM. Down syndrome: molecular mapping of the congenital heart disease and duodenal stenosis. *Am J Hum Genet.* 1992;50:294–302.
22. Van Praagh S, Truman T, Firpo A, et al. Cardiac malformations in trisomy-18: a study of 41 postmortem cases. *Am J Coll Cardiol.* 1989; 13:1586–1597.
23. Van Praagh S, Davidoff A, Chin A, Shiel FS, Reynolds J, Van Praagh R. Double-outlet right ventricle: anatomic types and developmental implications based on a study of 101 autopsied cases. *Coeur.* 1982;13: 389–439.
24. Van Praagh S, Santini F, Sanders SP. Cardiac malpositions with special emphasis on visceral heterotaxy (asplenia and polysplenia syndromes). In: Fyler DC, ed. *Nadas' Pediatric Cardiology.* Philadelphia: Hanley and Belfus; 1992:589–608.
25. Layton WM. Heart malformations in mice homozygous for a gene causing situs inversus. *Birth Defects.* (Orig Art Series) 1978;14:277–293.
26. Van Praagh R, Layton WM, Van Praagh S. The morphogenesis of normal and abnormal relationships between the great arteries and the ventricles: pathologic and experimental data. In: Van Praagh R, Takao A, eds. *Etiology and Morphogenesis of Congenital Heart Disease.* Mt Kisco, NY: Futura Publishing; 1980:271–316.
27. Brueckner M, D'Eustachio P, Horwich AL. Linkage mapping of a mouse gene, *iv,* that controls left-right asymmetry of the heart and viscera. *Proc Natl Acad Sci USA.* 1989;86:5035–5038.
28. Hanzlik AJ, Binder M, Layton WM, et al. The murine *situs inversus viscerum (iv)* gene responsible for visceral asymmetry is linked tightly to the *Igh-C* cluster on chromosome 12. *Genomics.* 1990;7:389–393.

CHAPTER *8*

HEART AND LUNG PATHOLOGY IN DOWN SYNDROME

Gaetano Thiene, Flavia Ventriglia, and Carla Frescura

NEARLY 40% OF PATIENTS WITH trisomy 21 (Down syndrome) present with a congenital heart disease (1,2). Atrioventricular septal defect ranks first, followed by isolated ventricular septal defect, ostium secundum atrial septal defect, and tetralogy of Fallot. Thus, congenital heart disease with left-to-right shunt prevails. Clinical and morphologic studies seem to support the view that patients with Down syndrome and left-to-right shunt malformations have a propensity to develop early and severe pulmonary vascular disease (3–5), but the matter is still controversial (6).

The aim of this chapter is first to report the incidence and types of congenital heart disease in specimens of our anatomic collection from patients with Down syndrome who died due to congenital heart disease and then to deal with the issue of pulmonary vascular disease, based on our experience with natural history, postoperative pathology, and lung biopsy. Other lung pathology in Down syndrome will also be reviewed.

Supported by the National Council for Research, Target Project "FAT.MA.," Rome, Italy.

Table 1. Cardiac registry of congenital heart disease: Sex and age distribution

Period	1967–1992
Number of specimens	970
Number of Down specimens	*67 (7%)*
Sex	37 males, 30 females
Age	2 days–11 years (median 4 months)

CARDIAC REGISTRY OF CONGENITAL HEART DISEASE AT THE UNIVERSITY OF PADUA

In the time period 1967–1992 we collected 970 heart–lung specimens with congenital heart disease. Sixty-seven (7%) belonged to patients with Down syndrome. Sex distribution was nearly equal (37 males, 30 females) and age varied from 2 days to 11 years (median 4 months) (Table 1).

Figure 1 displays the cumulative mortality according to age: 18% of patients with Down syndrome died within 1 month, 76% within 1 year, 94% within 5 years, and only 6% survived longer than 5 years. When compared with the survival of the overall population of autopsy cases with congenital heart disease, patients with Down syndrome had less mortality within 1 year and higher mortality in

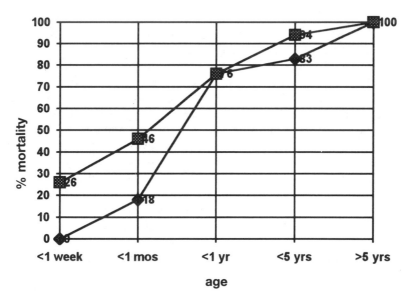

Figure 1. Cumulative mortality at the cardiac registry of congenital heart disease, University of Padua, 1967–1992. Patients with Down syndrome present with a lower mortality in the first months of life, and in the 1- to 5-year time interval have a higher mortality, probably as a result of the onset of pulmonary vascular disease. (——■—— = Overall population; ——♦—— = Patients with Down syndrome.)

the 1- to 5-year interval, probably because of onset of pulmonary vascular disease.

As far as the type of anomaly, only 3 of the 67 Down heart specimens presented with anomalous connections of cardiac segments: Two showed single aortic outlet in the setting of pulmonary atresia and one double-outlet right ventricle. The remaining 64 specimens basically showed normal connections of cardiac segments—namely, situs solitus, atrioventricular and ventriculoarterial concordance.

In Table 2, the major cardiac defects observed are listed. Atrioventricular septal defects come first (45 cases, 67%): isolated complete atrioventricular defect in 36, complete atrioventricular defect with tetralogy of Fallot in 7 and with double-outlet right ventricle in 1, and isolated partial atrioventricular defect in 1. Among the remaining 22 specimens (33%), isolated ventricular septal defect was observed in 6, isolated ostium secundum atrial septal defect in 6, tetralogy of Fallot in 3, pulmonary atresia with ventricular septal defect in 2, ventricular septal defect associated with aortic coarctation in 1 and with mitral cleft in 2, Ebstein's anomaly in 1, and patent ductus arteriosus in 1.

In Table 3 data of the cardiac registry concerning incidence and type of atrioventricular septal defects in Down versus non-Down specimens are reported. Among the 63 specimens with complete atrioventricular septal defect, 36 (57%) belonged to patients with

Table 2. Cardiac registry of congenital heart disease: Major cardiac defects

Atrioventricular septal defects		45 (67%)
Partial	1	
Complete	36	
Complete with TOF	7	
Complete with DORV	1	
Other defects (without atrioventricular septal defects)		22 (33%)
Isolated VSD	6	
VSD + mitral cleft	2	
VSD and aortic coarctation	1	
Isolated ASD secundum	6	
TOF	3	
Pulmonary atresia + VSD	1	
Pulmonary atresia + VSD + mitral cleft	1	
Ebstein	1	
Patent ductus	1	

Note: N = 67 patients.
ASD, atrial septal defect; DORV, double-outlet right ventricle; TOF, tetralogy of Fallot; VSD, ventricular septal defect.

Table 3. Cardiac registry of congenital heart disease: Incidence and type of atrio-ventricular septal defects

Anomaly	Down	Non-Down	Total
Isolated complete AV defect	36 (57%)	27 (43%)	63
Type A	18 (50%)	20 (74%)	
Type C	18 (50%)	7 (26%)	
Complete AV defect + TOF	7 (16%)	10 (27%)	17
Partial AV defect	1 (8%)	11 (92%)	12

AV, atrioventricular; TOF, tetralogy of Fallot.

Down syndrome and 27 (43%) to patients without Down syndrome; type C complete atrioventricular septal defect was more frequent in patients with Down syndrome than in the population with normal chromosomes. Association of complete atrioventricular canal with tetralogy of Fallot was observed in 16% of patients with Down syndrome and in 27% of patients without Down syndrome (p is not significant). Among the 12 specimens with partial atrioventricular septal defect, only 1 (8%) belonged to a patient with trisomy 21.

In summary, the above-mentioned figures, deriving from an autoptic population study, indicate the following:

1. Seven percent of patients with congenital heart disease present with a genetic background linked to Down syndrome.
2. The natural history shows high mortality of patients with Down syndrome within 5 years.
3. With very few exceptions, hearts from patients with Down syndrome exhibit a regular visceral symmetry and cardiac segment sequence.
4. Complete atrioventricular septal defect is the most common anomaly, having been observed in two thirds of specimens. Type C defect was more common in Down than in non–Down syndrome patients. The association of tetralogy of Fallot seems to be incidental (see Chapter 7).

PATHOLOGY OF THE LUNG IN DOWN SYNDROME

Patients with Down syndrome have problems not only at the cardiac level but also in the lungs. The latter may or may not be related to the heart defects. Following are the lung disorders:

1. Pulmonary vascular disease
2. Chronic upper airway obstruction
3. Pulmonary dysplasia
4. Pulmonary infections

PULMONARY VASCULAR DISEASE IN DOWN SYNDROME

There is still a controversy in the literature as to whether patients with Down syndrome have a propensity for early development of severe pulmonary vascular disease. In the late 1970s, we started to address the problem of determinants of failure in cardiac surgery of congenital heart disease (7). While studying the postoperative pathology of complete atrioventricular septal defect, we found that 4 of 15 patients, who died early after repair, presented a clinical picture of low cardiac output syndrome with pleural effusion, ascites, and liver congestion. All were affected by Down syndrome, 3 were younger than 1 year, and all exhibited a severe pulmonary vascular disease, with fibrinoid necrosis and glomoid and plexiform lesions (Figure 2). Surgical closure of the atrioventricular septal defect hindered the bidirectional shunt, thus creating an abrupt right ventricular pressure overload due to pulmonary hypertension (acute cor pulmonale). Pulmonary vascular lesions correlated well with the preoperative pulmonary vascular resistance values calculated during cardiac cath-

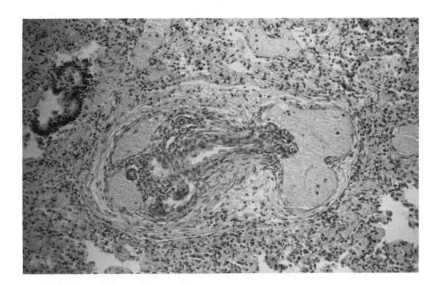

Figure 2.   A 3-year-old patient with Down syndrome and type C complete atrioventricular septal defect who died 4 hours after total repair surgery by a low output syndrome. Grade 4 pulmonary vascular disease with plexiform lesions was found at histology of the lungs (hematoxylin-eosin strain, original magnification ×40).

eterization. We concluded that advanced pulmonary vascular disease may interfere with the surgical outcome of atrioventricular septal defects even in infancy and that surgical correction should be anticipated.

Based on these preliminary data, we studied all the cases of our collection, with or without surgical repair, including a few lung biopsies performed at the time of surgery, with the aim of establishing the natural history of pulmonary vascular bed in patients with atrioventricular septal defects and to assess whether patients with Down syndrome have a true propensity for accelerated development of pulmonary vascular disease (8). Of the 49 patients, age ranging from 10 days to 14 years, median 9 months, 37 (75%) were affected by Down syndrome. The incidence of irreversible pulmonary vascular disease (Grade 3 or more) was 40.5% in Down syndrome versus 16% in patients without Down syndrome. Under 1 year of age, the most severe grades of pulmonary vascular disease (Grade 4) were seen in the time interval 7–12 months and only in patients with Down syndrome (Figure 3). These findings confirmed that the natural history of atrioventricular septal defects is characterized by early occurrence of pulmonary vascular disease, suggesting the need to perform surgical repair before the onset of irreversible lesions—namely, during the first months of life—and the propensity of the Down lungs to develop accelerated and severe vascular lesions.

In a following study, we investigated whether a lung biopsy may be useful for surgical decision making in congenital heart disease with left-to-right shunt, especially in patients in whom the hemodynamic findings do not provide a clear-cut picture or are borderline for surgery (9). The lung biopsies from 60 patients were studied, among which 25 had complete atrioventricular septal defect, 14 ventricular septal defect, and 7 complete transposition with ventricular septal defect. Age ranged from 3 months to 45 years, median 2 years. Twenty-one patients had Down syndrome, 18 in association with atrioventricular septal defect (Figure 4A) and 3 with ventricular septal defect (Figure 4B) (Table 4).

Irreversible lesions (equal to or greater than Grade 3) were observed in 30 cases (50%). Eight patients were younger than 1 year: 4 with atrioventricular defects (all Down) and 4 with complete transposition and ventricular septal defect (all without Down syndrome). Under 1 year of age, the more advanced lesions (Grade 4) were encountered in 1 patient with atrioventricular septal defect and Down syndrome and in the 4 patients with complete transposition and ventricular septal defect (Table 5). Thus, complete transposition and ventricular septal defect, even in the absence of Down syndrome, is

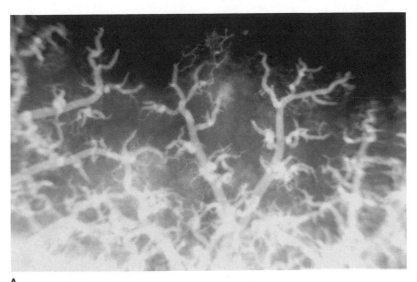

A

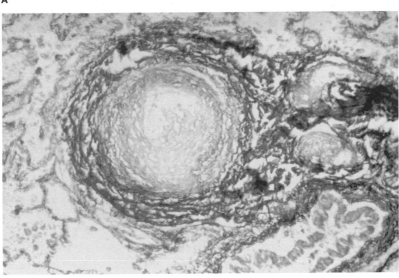

B

Figure 3. Obstructive pulmonary vascular disease in an 11-month-old infant with Down syndrome who died soon after surgery. **A:** X-ray of lungs after postmortem injection of contrast medium. Note the "winter tree" aspect of the pulmonary arterial vasculature. **B:** Lung histology exhibits severe obstructive vascular disease (Weigert–Van Gieson stain, original magnification ×40).

associated with a high propensity for accelerated and severe pulmonary vascular disease.

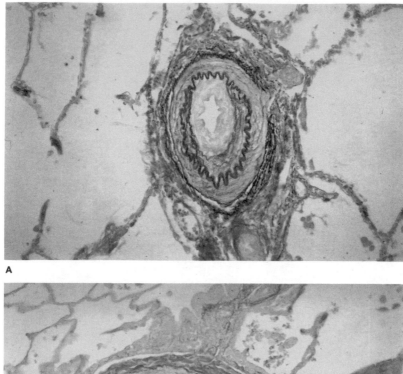

A

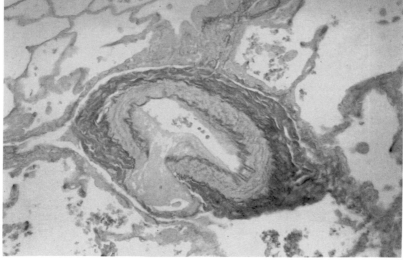

B

Figure 4. Lung biopsy. **A:** Grade 3 pulmonary vascular disease in a 4-year-old patient with Down syndrome and ventricular septal defect (Weigert–Van Gieson stain, original magnification ×50). **B:** Grade 4 pulmonary vascular disease in a 16-month-old infant with complete atrioventricular septal defect in Down syndrome (Weigert–Van Gieson stain, original magnification ×50).

Surgery was performed in 25 of the 30 patients with irreversible lesions (Table 6). The five nonoperated patients were still alive at the

Table 4. Lung biopsy in 60 cases of congenital heart disease: Distribution of lesions according to type of anomaly and histologic grading

Anomaly	No. cases	Histologic grading				
		0	1	2	3	4
AV septal defect	25[a]	1	11	2	9	2
VSD	14[b]	—	5	1	5	3
TGA and VSD	7	1	—	—	1	5
ASD	3	—	—	1	2	—
PDA	2	1	—	—	—	1
Others	9	3	4	—	2	—
Total	60	6	20	4	19	11

From (9) Frescura C, Thiene G, Franceschini E, et al. Is lung biopsy useful for surgical decision making in congenital heart disease? *Eur J Cardiothorac Surg.* 1991;5:118–123; Copyright © 1991 Springer-Verlag; reprinted with permission of Springer-Verlag.

[a]18 with Down syndrome.
[b]3 with Down syndrome.
Note: AV, atrioventricular; ASD, atrial septal defect; PDA, patent ductus arteriosus; TGA, transposition of the great arteries; VSD, ventricular septal defect.

time of study. Of the 25 operated patients, 10 (40%) died soon or at distance from intervention; the mortality was higher in Grade 3 patients (31%) than in Grade 4 patients (55%). Surgical outcome was particularly poor in those subjects with Grade 3–4 lesion who had persistent elevated pulmonary vascular resistance (>7 U/m^2) after oxygen administration at the time of hemodynamic study.

The conclusion of the study was that not only atrioventricular septal defect with Down syndrome but also complete transposition and ventricular septal defect in the absence of Down syndrome pre-

Table 5. Lung biopsy in congenital heart disease: Distribution of cases with "irreversible" lesions ($\geq$ Grade 3) according to age

Anomaly	Grade 3		Grade 4	
	<1 year	>1 year	<1 year	>1 year
AV septal defect	3	6	1[a]	1
VSD	—	5	—	3
TGA + VSD	—	1	4	1
ASD	—	2	—	—
PDA	—	—	—	1
Others	—	2	—	—
Total	3	16	5	6

From (9) Frescura C, Thiene G, Franceschini E, et al. Is lung biopsy useful for surgical decision making in congenital heart disease? *Eur J Cardiothorac Surg.* 1991;5:118–123; Copyright © 1991 Springer-Verlag; reprinted with permission of Springer-Verlag.

[a]With Down syndrome.
Note: ASD, atrial septal defect; AV, atrioventricular; PDA, patent ductus arteriosus; TGA, transposition of the great arteries; VSD, ventricular septal defect.

Table 6. Lung biopsy in congenital heart disease: Follow-up in 30 patients with Grade 3–4 pulmonary vascular disease

Category	Grade 3		Grade 4	
	Patients	Deaths	Patients	Deaths
Operated	16	5 (31%)	9	5 (55%)
Nonoperated	3	0	2	0
Total	19	5	11	5

From (9) Frescura C, Thiene G, Franceschini E, et al. Is lung biopsy useful for surgical decision making in congenital heart disease? *Eur J Cardiothorac Surg.* 1991;5:118–123; Copyright © 1991 Springer-Verlag; reprinted with permission of Springer-Verlag.

sents with a high propensity for accelerated and severe pulmonary vascular disease (9,10); lung biopsy is sensitive in detecting pulmonary vascular disease; the presence of irreversible lesions is predictive of severe, life-threatening pulmonary hypertension following surgical repair; and patients in such condition should be left unrepaired until progressive deterioration justifies cardiopulmonary transplantation.

CHRONIC UPPER AIRWAY OBSTRUCTION

Predisposition for accelerated pulmonary vascular disease in patients with Down syndrome, with and without congenital heart disease, has also been ascribed to chronic upper airway obstruction (see Chapter 11).

Structural abnormalities of the upper respiratory tract are often observed in patients with Down syndrome: a midfacial hypoplasia with short nasal passages, a narrowed hypopharynx, a small oral cavity, and mandibular and/or maxillary hypoplasia with a relative macroglossia and glossoptosis. Several airway abnormalities are also reported: choanal stenosis, hypertrophy of tonsils and adenoids, subglottic stenosis, tracheal narrowing, and laryngomalacia (11). Even chest wall abnormalities, such as pectum excavatum and carinatum with a weak thoracic musculature, contribute to cause chronic upper airway obstruction (11,12).

These obstructive lesions involving the upper airway result in chronic alveolar hypoventilation (13). The hypoventilation is usually most severe during sleep. The sleep-induced upper airway obstruction may be an important cause of accelerated pulmonary hypertension in patients with Down syndrome (14,15). The pathogenesis is multifactorial consisting of anatomic, functional, and neurologic difficulty (11). The anatomic features of Down syndrome added to muscular hypotonia may predispose to upper airway collapse during sleep, especially if enlargement of the tonsils and adenoids and nasal congestion are also present (14).

Obstructive apnea occurs when inspiratory airflow from the upper airway to the lungs is impeded for 10 seconds or greater, resulting in hypoxemia or hypercarbia. It happens most often during sleep when activation of pharyngeal dilator muscles decreases, thus causing relaxation of the airways; when the airway is exposed to negative pressure during the inspiratory effort, the airway collapse occurs (11).

The final common pathway for the sleep apnea and hypoventilation syndromes is a vasoconstrictive response of the pulmonary vascular bed to the chemical changes accompanying hypoventilation— that is, hypoxemia and hypercarbia with respiratory acidemia (13) (see Chapter 11).

PULMONARY DYSPLASIA IN DOWN SYNDROME

In the normal human fetus, the alveolar development does not begin until airway development is complete at 16 weeks. Between 4 and 6 months, the distal airway is transformed into a terminal respiratory bronchiole. Each respiratory bronchiole divides into three to six alveolar ducts. Each alveolar duct first ends in a terminal sac that ultimately evolves into definitive alveoli. The terminal respiratory unit shows a rapid increase during the first 2 years after birth (16,17).

Failure of the lung to develop properly either in the prenatal or the postnatal period has been proven to occur in patients with trisomy 21 and was presumed to be genetically determined. Different mechanisms of lung development have been postulated in Down syndrome (18,19). Cooney et al. (18) described abnormalities of the lungs in terms of both gross appearance and histologic evaluation. The peculiar gross appearance of the lungs in patients with Down syndrome consists of a diffuse and uniform porosity of the cut surface of the lungs due to enlargement of alveoli and alveolar ducts. Cooney et al. performed a radial alveolar count (20–22), which measures the average number of alveoli between terminal or respiratory bronchioles and the periphery of the acinus (so-called acinar complexity). A significantly diminished radial alveolar count (i.e., reduction in the alveoli number and a decrease in the alveoli surface) was calculated in the lungs of patients with Down syndrome, with or without congenital heart disease.

The gross appearance is due to the presence of dilated alveoli and alveolar ducts resulting from deficient alveolar multiplication (acinar hypoplasia) within the acinus. During the last period of gestation, the lungs presented with a normal alveolar count. The radial counts were noted to fall below normal in the immediate postnatal period, suggesting that this abnormality was acquired during the postnatal period. Decreased acinar complexity occurs and is grossly and microscopically apparent by 4 months of age. It persisted without change throughout childhood and adulthood. These abnormalities seem to be secondary to a lack of development rather than atrophy because of their lack of progression with age (18).

Thus, normal intrauterine lung growth may have different genetic control compared with normal postnatal growth. Intrauterine lung growth may be determined by maternal–placental factors and thus may be independent of fetus genetics. Alveolar formation is largely a postnatal, genetically controlled phenomenon.

In addition, Cooney et al. (18) observed a persistent alveolar double capillary network. It was considered as an integral part of the growth abnormality of the lung in Down syndrome. The abnormality consisted of a delicate alveolar wall with a central stroma of elastic tissue and parallel adjoining capillaries. It appears to be a separate, genetically determined defect. The alveolar double capillary network is a normal finding during intrauterine development. Normally an extensive remodeling occurs in the first year of life, whereas in Down syndrome this pattern remains during life, indicating failure of fusion of the two layers.

Schloo et al. (19) reached opposite conclusions by describing other patterns of disturbed lung growth in Down syndrome. They evaluated airway generations in a pulmonary segment by dissecting intrasegmental airway branches along several axial pathways. According to their findings, no single pattern can be considered characteristics of Down syndrome; airway branching is commonly reduced indicating impaired growth as early as the 10th to 12th week of intrauterine development; alveolar multiplication is also disturbed to such an extent as to yield a polyalveolar structure. This polyalveolar pattern is not simply a compensatory growth; this feature is found in the first days and months of postnatal life, indicating that it occurs antenatally. However, it is also apparent in older patients, suggesting that excessive multiplication can continue after birth.

The same mechanisms involved in the abnormal lung growth and cardiac development in patients with Down syndrome may also be involved in other parts of the body (19).

PULMONARY INFECTIONS

Mortality from respiratory infection has been reported to be 124 times higher in Down syndrome than in the general population (Figure 5) (23). The predisposition to infectious diseases in the respiratory tract is related to both structural and functional disorders and to

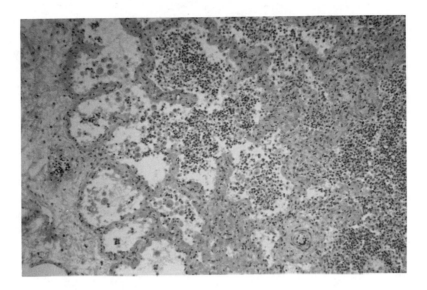

Figure 5. Fatal bronchopneumonia in a 4-year-old patient with Down syndrome and complete atrioventricular septal defect. Note the alveolar essudate (hematoxylin-eosin stain, original magnification ×30).

cellular and/or humoral immunodefects associated with Down syndrome (11).

The pulmonary infections are one of the major causes of morbidity and mortality throughout the various age groups. Sinus infections may often be the antecedent infection to lower respiratory tract illness because of a reduced mucociliary clearance. In patients with Down syndrome signs and symptoms of pulmonary infection can be more acute than in the general population. Bacterial pneumonia is common and is associated with fever and leukocytosis. The primary organisms are *Staphylococcus aureus* and *Hemophilus influenzae* (24). Viral infections such as respiratory syncytial virus, parainfluenza virus, and adenoinfluenza virus may also present with acute respiratory distress and significant morbidity (25).

The propensity for infections of the lower respiratory tract can be explained in terms of pulmonary congestion due to congenital heart disease with a large left-to-right shunt (see Chapter 13). The increased work of breathing is secondary to the added inflammation and edema of the airways superimposed on a chronic state of increased interstitial fluid. Moreover, the enlargement of heart chambers and great arteries causes compression of the left bronchus. In Down syndrome, aspiration and/or gastroesophageal reflux also recurs due to an increased incidence of esophageal dysfunction (26), with ab ingestis pneumonia.

Clinical and laboratory evidence suggests that immunodeficiency is an integral feature of Down syndrome (27). These subjects have a deficiency of both cell- and antibody-mediated immunity. A selective T-cell defect, with a significant reduction of CD3+, CD1+, CD4+, and CD8+ cells and an inversion of CD4/CD8 (28), could be the primary event in Down syndrome. In fact, in thymuses of patients with Down syndrome there is a deficient expansion of immature T cells, resulting in a reduction of the various thymocyte subpopulations (28). This event disturbs the immune homeostasis and increases risk of malignancies since the first few years of life. Repeated infections that depress the immune function cause a "stress deficiency" of the immune system leading to precocious aging of both cell-mediated and antibody-mediated immunity (27).

REFERENCES

1. Spicer RL. Cardiovascular disease in Down syndrome. *Pediatr Clin North Am.* 1984;31:1331–1343.
2. Marino B. Cardiac aspects. In: Pueschel SM, Pueschel JK, eds. *Biomedical Concerns in Persons with Down Syndrome.* Baltimore: Paul H. Brookes Publishing Co.; 1992:91–105.
3. Soudon P, Stijns M, Tremourox-Wattiez M, Vliers A. Precocity of pulmonary vascular obstruction in Down's syndrome. *Eur J Cardiol.* 1975; 2/4:473–476.
4. Chi TPL, Krovetz J. The pulmonary vascular bed in children with Down syndrome. *J Pediatr.* 1975;86:533–538.
5. Clapp S, Perry BL, Farooki ZQ, et al. Down's syndrome, complete atrioventricular canal, and pulmonary vascular obstructive disease. *J Thorac Cardiovasc Surg.* 1990;100:115–121.
6. Plett JA, Tandon R, Moller JH, Edwards JE. Hypertensive pulmonary vascular disease. *Arch Pathol.* 1974;97:187–188.
7. Thiene G, Mazzucco A, Franceschini E, et al. Postoperative pathology of complete atrioventricular defects. *J Thorac Cardiovasc Surg.* 1982; 83:891–900.
8. Frescura C, Thiene G, Franceschini E, Talenti E, Mazzucco A. Pulmonary vascular disease in infants with complete atrioventricular septal defect. *Int J Cardiol.* 1987;15:91–100.
9. Frescura C, Thiene G, Gagliardi MG, et al. Is lung biopsy useful for surgical decision making in congenital heart disease? *Eur J Cardiothorac Surg.* 1991;5:118–123.
10. Yamaki S, Horiuchi T, Sekino Y. Quantitative analysis of pulmonary vascular disease in simple cardiac anomalies with the Down syndrome. *Am J Cardiol.* 1983;51:1502–1506.
11. Howenstine MS. Pulmonary concerns. In: Pueschel SM, Pueschel JK, eds. *Biomedical Concerns in Persons with Down Syndrome.* Baltimore: Paul H. Brookes Publishing Co.; 1992:105–118.

12. Rowland TW, Nordstrom LG, Bean MS, Burkhardt H. Chronic upper airway obstruction and pulmonary hypertension in Down's syndrome. *Am J Dis Child.* 1981;135:1050–1052.
13. Levine OR, Simpser M. Alveolar hypoventilation and cor pulmonale associated with chronic airway obstruction in infants with Down syndrome. *Clin Pediatr.* 1982;21:25–29.
14. Loughlin GM, Wynne JW, Victorica BE. Sleep apnea as a possible cause of pulmonary hypertension in Down syndrome. *J Pediatr.* 1981; 98:435–437.
15. Marcus CL, Keens TG, Bautista DB, Von Pechmann WS, Ward SL. Obstructive sleep apnea in children with Down syndrome. *Pediatrics.* 1991;88:132–139.
16. Netter FH. In: Divertie MB, Brass A, eds. *The ABE Collection of Medical Illustrations. Vol. 7: Respiratory System.* CIBA, 1979;7:39–40.
17. Thurlbeck WM. Postnatal human lung growth. *Thorax.* 1982;37: 564–571.
18. Cooney TP, Wentworth PJ, Thurlbeck WM. Diminished radial count is found only postnatally in Down's syndrome. *Ped Pulmonol.* 1988;5: 204–209.
19. Schloo BL, Vawter GF, Reid LM. Down syndrome: patterns of disturbed lung growth. *Hum Pathol.* 1991;22:919–923.
20. Emery JL, Mithal A. The number of alveoli in the terminal respiratory unit of man during late intrauterine life and childhood. *Arch Dis Child.* 1960;35:544–547.
21. Cooney TP, Thurlbeck WM. The radial alveolar count method of Emery and Mithal: a reappraisal 1–Postnatal lung growth. *Thorax.* 1982;37: 572–579.
22. Cooney TP, Thurlbeck WM. The radial alveolar count method of Emery and Mithal: a reappraisal 2—Intrauterine and early postnatal lung growth. *Thorax.* 1982;37:580–583.
23. Oster J, Mikkelsen M, Nielsen A. Mortality and life-table in Down's syndrome. *Acta Paediatr Scand.* 1975;64:322.
24. Cant AJ, Gibson PJ, West RJ. Bacterial tracheitis in Down's syndrome. *Arch Dis Child.* 1987;62:962–963.
25. Wohl ME. Bronchiolitis. *Pediatrics.* 1985;15:307–313.
26. Hillemeier C, Buchin PJ, Gryboski J. Esophageal dysfunction in Down's syndrome. *J Ped Gastroenterol Nutr.* 1982;1:101–104.
27. Ugazio AG, Lanzavecchia A, Jayakar S, Plebani A, Duse M, Burgio R. Immunodeficiency in Down's syndrome. *Acta Paediatr Scand.* 1978; 67:705–708.
28. Musiani P, Valitutti S, Castellino F, Larocca LM, Maggiano N, Piantelli M. Intrathymic deficient expansion of T cell precursors in Down syndrome. *Am J Med Genet.* 1990;7(suppl):219–224.

—————— CHAPTER *9* ——————

CARDIOVASCULAR MANIFESTATIONS IN PERSONS WITH DOWN SYNDROME

M. Quero Jimenez,
M.J. Maitre Azcarate,
and M.C. Manrique

Down SYNDROME TRISOMY 21 IS the most frequently identified chromosome abnormality in liveborn infants (1). It occurs once among 650 live newborns and once among 22 patients with congenital heart disease. Down syndrome is the most frequent polimalformative complex in pediatric cardiology services. There is no predilection for either sex. In relation to mother age, it is more frequent above 35 and below 20 years.

Generally speaking, cardiovascular malformations in Down syndrome may be cardiac or vascular, congenital or acquired, and all in all affect approximately 60% of the population with this aneuploidy. By far, congenital heart defects are more frequent, accounting for approximately 55% of individuals with Down syndrome. Pulmonary vasculature involvement is noted frequently, with its basis probably being both congenital and acquired.

CONGENITAL HEART DEFECTS

The frequency of congenital heart defects in children with Down syndrome is roughly 50%, which is probably an underestimate, considering that cases of intrauterine death, spontaneous abortion, and minimal congenital heart disease are not usually included in most series.

The most frequent cardiac malformations in Down syndrome are usually acyanotic and are characterized by huge left-to-right intra-cardiac shunts at both the atrial and/or the ventricular level. Extra-cardiac shunts, such as persistent ductus arteriosus, may exist but are not common when isolated. Other acyanotic cardiac defects in Down syndrome, such as left-sided obstructive and/or valvular lesions and vascular rings, are very uncommon (Table 1). The incidence of cy-anotic heart defects, excluding Eisenmenger, is approximately 10%, most of them corresponding to patients with tetralogy of Fallot, either associated to complete atrioventricular septal defect (atrioventricular canal) or isolated. Double-outlet/double-inlet ventricles plus pulmo-nary stenosis or atresia, so common in Ivemark syndrome, are ex-ceedingly rare in Down syndrome. Indeed, well-documented cases with complete transposition of the great arteries are exceptional (Ta-ble 1).

The complete form of atrioventricular canal is the most common and characteristic cardiac defect in patients with Down syndrome. Atrioventricular canal is usually characterized by a common atrio-ventricular annulus and orifice extending from one ventricle to the other through the middle of a huge septal atrioventricular defect, re-sulting from contiguous and committed atrial and ventricular septal defects. The atrioventricular septal defect in patients with Down syn-

Table 1. Down syndrome: Cardiovascular malformations in 415 patients

Malformation	Incidence (%)
Acyanotic: Left-to-right shunts	
Atrioventricular septal defects	52
Ventricular septal defects	26
Patent ductus arteriosus	4
Atrial septal defect	3
Cyanotic: Right-to-left or bidirectional shunts	
Tetralogy of Fallot	9
Double-outlet ventricle	0.8
Obstructions of the left heart and valvular malformations	
Isolated mitral abnormalities	2
Isolated aortic coarctation	1.5
Isolated aortic valvar stenosis	0.3
Vascular anomalies	
Anomalous retroesophageal subclavian artery	11.5

drome usually corresponds to Rastelli Type C (2) in which the presence of a large, anterior, bridging leaflet has been interpreted as a very primitive faulty development of the atrioventricular cushions and surrounding tissues (3). Ventricular volumes and masses are well balanced in individuals with Down syndrome compared with patients with Ivemark syndrome (4) and with those with normal chromosomes (5).

Clinically, heart failure and severe respiratory complications appear around 1 month of age or even earlier, when associated obstructive abnormalities of the systemic circulation coexist. Pulmonary vascular disease occurs early on and is severe in nature. This has been partly attributed to hypoventilation resulting from facial abnormalities involving narrowed airways and hypoplasia of the lung, with poor bronchial and pulmonary artery branching (6,7,8). Partial forms of atrioventricular septal defect, such as ostium primum, may exist but are rare (5). The morphology of the defects is the same when associated with the infundibular abnormalities that characterize tetralogy of Fallot. The clinical picture then is that of cyanosis and cyanotic attacks appearing at different ages and with different severity according to the degree of right ventricular infundibular obstruction.

The second most common heart malformation in Down syndrome is ventricular septal defect. Manifestations of large ventricular septal defects resemble those of atrioventricular septal defects. Morphologically, the defect is perimembranous and extends to the inlet septum more frequently than in ventricular septal defects of persons who do not have Down syndrome (9).

POSTOPERATIVE PROBLEMS

Postoperative problems do not differ very much from the usual postoperative complications of infants with severe congenital heart disease in general. They can be divided into early and late complications; both are related to the particular location of conducting tissue and to the anatomical and functional features of the pulmonary circulation.

The proximity of the conducting tissue to the superior rim of the ventricular septum was the origin of the increased frequency of atrioventricular block at the beginning of surgical correction of atrioventricular septal defects. With increased progressive surgical skill, this complication is now rare. Nevertheless it is still advisable to leave epicardial electrodes to be used in case of the occurrence of an atrioventricular block, even if transient in nature. Other early postoperative dysrhythmias, such as perioperative trivial nodal tachycardia, are well tolerated and self-limited, usually disappearing spontaneously.

The anatomic and functional derangements of pulmonary circulation in patients with Down syndrome resulting in development of early and particularly severe pulmonary vascular disease often lead to postoperative pulmonary hypertensive crisis, the management of which is based on prevention and treatment. These crises often result in profound deterioration and even death and are usually triggered by agitation following suctioning of bronchial secretions, hypoxia, hypothermia, hypoglycemia, hypocalcemia, acidosis, polycythemia, and alterations in the electrolyte pattern.

Even cardiopulmonary bypass itself may be a precipitating feature through platelet damage, resulting in abnormal production of vasoconstrictive substances, the origin of which may be the vascular endothelium. Many of these precipitating features may be controlled by appropriate and careful handling of the patient. In ventilating patients with Down syndrome and congenital heart defects presenting with increased pulmonary blood flow and generalized bronchial and pulmonary vascular hypoplasia, it should be kept in mind that the compliance of the lungs is significantly reduced and that the advantages of being ventilated with positive and expiratory pressure have to be matched with reduction of cardiac output. Hyperventilation–respiratory alkalosis is a good means of both preventing and treating crises of pulmonary hypertension. Paralysis with pancuronium, reducing handling to a minimal and experienced one, and correcting acidosis, electrolyte deviations, and hypothermia are all necessary measures. Careful tracheal suctioning should be performed only when necessary and preceded by an intravenous bolus injection of fentanyl (30 μg/kg). As pulmonary vasodilator drugs, prostaglandins E_1, nitroprusside, phenoxybenzamine, and prostacycline are useful when administrated at an appropriate dosage. Even after discharge, pulmonary pressure should be carefully evaluated during long-term follow-up.

In conclusion, some excellent results have been achieved in the correction of severe congenital heart defects such as tetralogy of Fallot and complete atrioventricular septal defect (9,10) in children with Down syndrome.

REFERENCES

1. LeJeune J, Turpin R. Chromosomal aberrations in man. *Am J Hum Genet.* 1961;13:175–188.
2. Rastelli GC, Kirklin JW, Titus JL. Anatomic observations on complete form of persistent common atrioventricular canal with special reference to atrioventricular valves. *Mayo Clin Proc.* 1966;41:246–308.

3. Ugarte M, Enriquez de Salamanca F, Quero Jimenez M. Endocardial cushion defects. An anatomical study of 54 specimens. *Br Heart J.* 1976;38:674–682.
4. Cabrera A, Quero Jimenez M, Pastor E, et al. Asplenia y polisplenia. Estudio anatomico de 27 casos y revision de la literatura. *Rev Lat Cardiol.* 1981;2:83–89.
5. Marino B, Vairo U, Corno A, Nava S, Guccione P, Calabrò R, Marcelletti C. Atrioventricular canal in Down syndrome. Prevalence of associated cardiac malformations compared with patients without Down syndrome. *Am J Dis Child.* 1990;144:1120–1122.
6. Yamaki S, Horiuchi T, Takahashi T. Pulmonary changes in congenital heart disease with Down syndrome. Their significance as a cause of postoperative respiratory failure. *Thorax.* 1985;40:380–386.
7. Cooney TP, Thurlbeck WM. Pulmonary hypoplasia in Down's syndrome. *N Engl J Med.* 1982;307(19):1170–1173.
8. Marino B, Papa M, Guccione P, Corno A, Marasini M, Calabrò R. Ventricular septal defect in Down syndrome: anatomic type and associated malformations. *Am J Dis Child.* 1990;144:544–545.
9. Alonso J, Nunez P, Perez de Leon J, et al. Complete atrioventricular canal and tetralogy of Fallot. Surgical management. *Eur J Cardiothorac Surg.* 1990;4:297–303.
10. DaSilva AE, Maitre MJ, Sanchez PA, Quero Jimenez M, Brito JM, Vellibre D. Defecto del septo atrioventricular con tetralogia de Fallot. Aspectos clinicomorfologicos y consideraciones quirurgicas. *Rev Esp Cardiol.* 1989;42:597–604.

—————— CHAPTER *10*——————

PATTERNS OF CONGENITAL HEART DISEASE AND ASSOCIATED CARDIAC ANOMALIES IN CHILDREN WITH DOWN SYNDROME

Bruno Marino

THE STUDY OF VARIOUS TYPES of congenital heart defects in children with Down syndrome has long attracted the attention of researchers. The association between Mongolian idiocy and defects of the interauricular septum, especially ostium primum or patent atrioventricularis communis, had already been reported by Maud Abbot (1924) and Helen Taussig (1947) in their pioneer studies.

Moreover, in concluding his study *Cardiac Anomalies in Mongolism*, published by the *British Heart Journal* in 1950 (1), Philip Evans wrote

Congenital heart disease was found in nearly half of mongol imbeciles dying in the first five years of life. In the records of 63 autopsies of persons with Down syndrome 28 had congenital heart disease. Ventricular and atrial septal defect each accounted for one third of the individual lesions and patent ductus arteriosus for one sixth. Pulmonary stenosis and persistent atrioventricularis communis each occurred in four patients. Compared with children with congenital heart disease dying in the same hospital during the same time period, transposition of the great vessels, coarctation, and truncus arteriosus seemed to be unassociated with mongolism. (p. 260)

Numerous studies (2–11) have since confirmed that children with trisomy 21 present certain congenital heart defects and seem to be *protected* from others. It is currently ascertained that infants with Down syndrome are at 40%–50% risk for congenital heart defects. The most often observed cardiac lesions are atrioventricular canal (60% of all diseases), ventricular septal defect, tetralogy of Fallot, patent ductus arteriosus, and atrial septal defect (2–11).

Other anomalies, such as isolated pulmonary valve stenosis or atresia, aortic valve stenosis or atresia, and aortic coarctation, are rare. Moreover, some heart defects are virtually absent, such as anomalies of the visceroatrial situs, ventricular inversion (L loop), atresia of the atrioventricular valves, double-inlet left ventricle with two separate valves, truncus arteriosus, and transposition of the great arteries.

However, in Chinese (12) and Mexican (13) patients with Down syndrome the frequency of various types of congenital heart diseases seems different. In agreement with the genetic similarities of these two populations (14), the most common cardiac defect in Chinese and Mexican children with Down syndrome is ventricular septal defect followed by atrioventricular canal (12,13). These data suggest that in these persons with Down syndrome other genetic or environmental factors may be involved in the pathogenesis of the various types of congenital heart disease.

Interestingly, although Down syndrome is more common in males (15), females more often have associated congenital heart disease (11,16). The explanation for this prevalence or rarity of heart disease and for this different distribution between the sexes is not known.

At the beginning of our research on congenital heart defects in children with Down syndrome, we asked ourselves the following questions:

1. Do morphologic peculiarities of the more frequently observed congenital heart defects in patients with Down syndrome exist in comparison to those with normal chromosomes?
2. Do children with trisomy 21 who do not have congenital heart defects present a completely normal cardiac anatomy?
3. What is the prevalence and what are the types of congenital heart diseases in children with mosaicism Down syndrome?

From 1982 to 1992 we studied 481 children with Down syndrome, 381 with and 100 without congenital heart defect (17). The cardiac malformations are summarized in Table 1. The morphologic diagnosis resulted from echocardiographic and angiocardiographic studies as well as from surgical reports or postmortem data. The anatomic characteristics of these patients and the prevalence of associated cardiac anomalies were compared to those of chromosomally normal children with the same type of heart defect and same age. Statistical analysis was then performed.

ATRIOVENTRICULAR CANAL

The complete form of atrioventricular canal is most commonly associated with Down syndrome. Among all of our patients, 70% with complete atrioventricular canal have trisomy 21. However, the partial form of atrioventricular canal was more prevalent in children with normal chromosomes (75% of our cases) (18). Among those with complete atrioventricular canal, Rastelli Type C (19) is rarest in patients who do not have Down syndrome. Associated cardiac anomalies are significantly more frequent in patients without Down syndrome: 70% of these additional anomalies occur in patients with atrioventricular canal and normal chromosomes and only 30% in children with Down syndrome.

In patients with trisomy 21, the only prevalent associated malformation is tetralogy of Fallot. In our experience, it is present in 18% of patients with complete atrioventricular canal and Down syndrome and in only 10% of chromosomally normal patients (18). However, children with complete atrioventricular canal who do not have Down syndrome have a very high prevalence (65%) of other types of associated cardiac anomalies. These include muscular ventricular septal defect (20), malformation of the mitral valve, hypoplasia of the left ventricle with right ventricular dominance (21), and coarctation of the aorta. In addition, patients with the partial form and normal chromosomes are at higher risk for left-sided cardiac anomalies such as the mitral valve as well as of the left ventricular inlet and outlet tracts (18,21,22). On the contrary, left ventricular dominance with hypoplasia of the right ventricle may occur in children

Table 1. Incidence of cardiac malformations among children with Down syndrome

Malformation	Number of cases	Percent
Atrioventricular canal	229	60
Ventricular septal defect	121	32
Tetralogy of Fallot	25	6
Atrial septal defect	3	1
Isolated mitral cleft	3	1

with complete atrioventricular canal and Down syndrome, sometimes associated with tetralogy of Fallot. This association of defects is rarest in patients with normal chromosomes.

In conclusion, children with Down syndrome show a simple type of atrioventricular canal, usually complete, rarely associated with other cardiac anomalies (except tetralogy of Fallot) (18). Particularly rare are the left-sided anomalies, which are more frequent in patients with atrioventricular canal and normal chromosomes (21). Genes located on different chromosomes could be responsible for atrioventricular canal in patients without Down syndrome.

VENTRICULAR SEPTAL DEFECT

In children with Down syndrome a posterior perimembranous ventricular septal defect in the inlet segment of the ventricular septum is frequently observed (30% of our patients with Down syndrome vs. 4% in patients without trisomy 21) (23). Muscular and subarterial ventricular septal defects are rare in trisomy 21. Among the additional anomalies, the only prevalent association with Down syndrome is the cleft of the mitral valve (20% in children with Down syndrome vs. 1% without Down syndrome). In contrast, left ventricular outflow tract obstruction (17% without Down syndrome vs. 1% with Down syndrome) is prevalent in children with normal chromosomes (23). Moreover, mitral stenosis and tricuspid straddling are very rare in patients with Down syndrome who have ventricular septal defect. Inlet ventricular septal defect with a cleft of the mitral valve is frequent in patients with Down syndrome and represents a link with the persistent atrioventricular canal. These results on ventricular septal defect confirm the rarity of left ventricular inlet and outlet obstruction previously reported in children with Down syndrome as isolated anomalies (1–11,24) and with major heart defects (21,25). Furthermore, although defects in the perimembranous septum are frequently seen in children with Down syndrome (isolated ventricular septal defect, atrioventricular canal, tetralogy of Fallot), the trabecular muscular ventricular septal defect is rare as an isolated anomaly (22) and in association with major defects (20–26). This segment of ventricular septum, frequently affected in cases with aortic coarctation, seems to be *protected* in children with Down syndrome. These data about atrioventricular canal and ventricular septal defect (27,28) were recently confirmed in a large epidemiologic investigation by the Baltimore and Washington Infant Study Group (24,29). We do not know why these anatomic differences occur. They could be explained on the basis of intrinsic genetic mechanisms and/or of alterations in embryonic blood flow patterns (30).

TETRALOGY OF FALLOT

Tetralogy of Fallot is the only contruncal anomaly occurring in children with Down syndrome. In patients with trisomy 21, tetralogy of Fallot is usually an isolated finding, and the only additional cardiovascular anomaly associated is atrioventricular canal sometimes with hypoplastic right ventricle (18). Other cardiac malformations, such as pulmonary atresia, absent pulmonary valve, absent infundibular septum, and discontinuity of the pulmonary arteries, sometimes observed in association with tetralogy of Fallot in patients with normal chromosomes or in patients with deletion of chromosome 22 are exceptionally rare in children with tetralogy of Fallot and Down syndrome.

With regard to additional chromosomal errors, we recently observed another patient with atrioventricular canal, mosaicism trisomy 21, and Turner syndrome (45,x/46,xx,i[21q]) (31).

CARDIAC GEOMETRY IN CHILDREN WITH DOWN SYNDROME WITHOUT CONGENITAL HEART DISEASE

The cardiac anatomy in persons with trisomy 21 without congenital heart disease is supposed to be normal. However, there are no specific data supporting this assumption. In our echocardiography study of 100 children with Down syndrome without congenital heart disease, we measured the interatrial septum length, the systolic and diastolic left ventricular dimensions, the offsetting of atrioventricular valves, and the inlet and outlet dimensions of the left ventricle (32). Comparing these data to those of a control group of chromosomally normal children, we found an elongation of the left ventricular outflow dimension in patients with Down syndrome, whereas the inlet dimension was similar in the two groups. Moreover, we noted a tendency toward the insertion of the atrioventricular valves at the same level of the ventricular septum. Thus, even in the absence of congenital heart disease, persons with Down syndrome may have asymptomatic abnormal cardiac structures. These echocardiographic results correspond to the previous anatomic observations of enlargement of the membranous ventricular septum reported by Rosenquist (33,34). These morphologic aberrations may represent a subclinical internal phenotype of the heart in persons with Down syndrome (28). Thus, individuals with Down syndrome present not only the specific type of atrioventricular canal and ventricular septal defect, but also peculiar, minor structural abnormalities of the normal heart.

CONGENITAL HEART DISEASE IN MOSAICISM DOWN SYNDROME

Because no other studies exist in the literature on the prevalence and types of congenital heart disease in patients with mosaicism trisomy 21, we analyzed by echocardiography 27 unselected patients with mosaicism Down syndrome (34).

Only eight patients (29.6%) had congenital heart disease: four had atrioventricular canal (one complete and three partial), two had ventricular septal defects, one had atrial septal defect, and one had patent ductus arteriosus. Our results suggest a lower prevalence and less severity of congenital heart disease in subjects with mosaicism Down syndrome (36) when compared with equivalent data of congenital heart disease in patients with complete trisomy 21 (1–11). We postulate that phenotypic expression at the cardiac level is less severe in these individuals. These findings may be explained on the basis of the partial aneuploidy itself or of a tissue-specific localization in mosaicism Down syndrome.

In conclusion, we can state that from an anatomic point of view the *pattern* of congenital heart disease in patients with Down syndrome is not worse than that observed in patients with normal chromosomes. Furthermore, cardiac malformations of subjects with Down syndrome are less complex and more predictable. Therefore, surgical results in this group of patients are similar and sometimes even better than those achieved in patients with the same heart defect who do not have chromosome anomalies (37–41).

REFERENCES

1. Evans PR. Cardiac anomalies in mongolism. *Br Heart J.* 1950;12: 258–262.
2. Liu MC, Corlett K. A study of congenital heart defects in mongolism. *Arch Dis Child.* 1959;12:410–419.
3. Berg JM, Crome L, France NE. Congenital cardiac malformations in mongolism. *Br Heart J.* 1960;22:331–346.
4. Rowe RD, Uchida IA. Cardiac malformation in mongolism. *Am J Med.* 1961;31:726–735.
5. Rowe RD. Cardiac malformation in mongolism. *Am Heart J.* 1962;64: 567–569.
6. Warkany J, Passarge E, Smith LB. Congenital malformations in autosomal trisomy syndromes. *Am J Dis Child.* 1966;112:502–517.
7. Cullum L, Liebman J. The association of congenital heart disease with Down's syndrome (mongolism). *Am J Med.* 1969;24:354–357.

8. Tandon R, Edwards JE. Cardiac malformations associated with Down's syndrome. *Circulation.* 1973;47:1349–1355.
9. Laursen HB. Congenital heart disease in Down's syndrome. *Br Heart J.* 1976;38:32–38.
10. Greenwood RD, Nadas AS. The clinical course of cardiac disease in Down's syndrome. *Pediatrics.* 1976;58:893–897.
11. Park SC, Mathews RA, Zuberbuhler JR, Rowe RD, Neches WH, Lenox CC. Down syndrome with congenital heart malformation. *Am J Dis Child.* 1977;131:29–33.
12. Sing Roxy LN, Maurice LP, Chiu LK, Yung YC. Congenital cardiovascular malformations in Chinese children with Down syndrome. *Clin Med J.* 1989;102/5:382–386.
13. Vizcaino V. Personal communication, Mexico City, 1993.
14. Cavalli Sforza LL, Menozzi P, Piazza A. Demic expansions and human evolution. *Science.* 1993;259:639–646.
15. Fabia J, Drolette M. Life tables up to age 10 for mongols with and without congenital heart disease. *J Ment Defic Res.* 1970;14:235–242.
16. Pinto FF, Nunes L, Ferraz F, Sanpayo F. Down's syndrome: different distribution of congenital heart disease between the sexes. *Int J Cardiol.* 1990;27:175–178.
17. Digilio MC, Marino B, Giannotti A, Dallapiccola B. Familial atrioventricular septal defect. *Br Heart J.* In press.
18. Marino B, Vairo U, Corno A, Nava S, Guccione P, Calabrò R, Marcelletti C. Atrioventricular canal in Down syndrome. *Am J Dis Child.* 1990; 144:1120–1122.
19. Rastelli GC, Kirklin JW, Titus JL. Anatomic observations on complete form of persistent common atrioventricular canal with special reference to atrioventricular valves. *Mayo Clin Proc.* 1966;41:296–308.
20. Papa M, Marino B, Vairo U, Nava S, Parretti di Iulio D, Donfrancesco C, Cicini MP, Grazioli S, Mazzera E, Marcelletti C. Difetto interventricolare muscolare nel canale atrioventricolare. *G Ital Cardiol.* 1990; 20:801–804.
21. De Biase L, Di Ciommo L, Ballerini L, Bevilacqua M, Marcelletti C, Marino B. Prevalence of left-sided obstruction lesion in patients with atrioventricular canal without Down's syndrome. *J Thorac Cardiovasc Surg.* 1986;91:467–472.
22. Giamberti A, Marino B, Di Donato R, Grazioli S, Marcelletti C. Canale atrioventricolare parziale: fattori di deterioramento clinico e risultati chirurgici nel primo anno di vita. *G Ital Cardiol.* 1990;20:19.
23. Marino B, Papa M, Guccione P, Corno A, Marasini M, Calabrò R. Ventricular septal defect in Down syndrome. Anatomic types and associated malformation. *Am J Dis Child.* 1990;144:544–545.
24. Ferencz C, Neill CA, Boughman JA. Congenital cardiovascular malformations with chromosome abnormalities: an epidemiologic study. *J Pediatr.* 1989;144:79–86.
25. Marino B. Left sided cardiac obstruction in patients with Down syndrome. *J Pediatr.* 1989;115:834–835.
26. Marino B, Corno A, Guccione P, Marcelletti C. Ventricular septal defect and Down's syndrome. *Lancet.* 1991;337:245–246.
27. Marino B. Cardiac aspects. In: Pueschel SM, Pueschel JK, eds., *Biomedical Concerns in Persons with Down Syndrome.* Baltimore: Paul H. Brookes Publishing Co.; 1992:91–103.

28. Marino B. Atrioventricular septal defect. Anatomic characteristics in patients with and without Down's syndrome. *Cardiol Young.* 1992;2: 308–310.

29. Ferencz C, Carmi R, Bougham JA. Endocardial cushion defect: further studies of "isolated" versus "syndromic" occurrence. *Am J Med Genet.* 1992;43:569–575.

30. Genarelli M, Novelli G, Digilis MC, Giannotti A, Marino B, Dellapiccola B. *Hum Genet.*1994;94:708–710.

31. Digilio MC, Mingarelli R, Marino B, Giannotti A, Melchionda S, Dallapiccola B. Congenital cardiac defect in a patient with mosaic 45,X/ 46,XX,i(21q) karyotype. *Clin Genet.* 1994;46:268–270.

32. Annicchiarico M, Marino B, Ammirati A, Affinito V, Di Carlo D, Ragonese P. Is cardiac anatomy in children with Down's syndrome without congenital heart disease "normal"? An echocardiographic study. *Circulation.* 1992;86:I-571.

33. Rosenquist CG, Sweeney BA, Amsel J, MacAllister HA. Enlargement of the membranous ventricular septum: an internal stigma of Down's syndrome. *J Pediatr.* 1974;85:490–493.

34. Rosenquist GC, Sweeney BA, MacAllister H. A relationship of the tricuspid valve to the membranous ventricular septum in Down's syndrome without endocardial cushion defect: study of 28 specimens, 14 with a ventricular septal defect. *J Pediatr.* 1975;90:458–462.

35. De Zorzi A, Marino B, Milanesi O, Calabrò R, Marasini M, Santilli A, Parretti di Iulio D. Cardiopatie congenite nella sindrome di Down con mosaicismo: risultati preliminari. *G Ital Cardiol.* 1991;21:31.

36. Marino B, De Zorzi A. Congenital heart disease in trisomy 21 mosaicism. *J Pediatr.* 1993;122(3):500–501.

37. Schneider DS, Zahka KG, Clark EB, Neill CA. Patterns of cardiac care in infants with Down syndrome. *Am J Dis Child.* 1989;143:363–365.

38. Vet TW, Ottenkamp J. Correction of atrioventricular septal defect. *Am J Dis Child.* 1989;143:1361–1365.

39. Williams WH, Perrella AM, Plauth WH, Hatcher CR, Guyton RA. Survival following repair of complete atrioventricular canal associated with Down's syndrome. In: Crupi GC, Parenzan L, Anderson RH, eds. *Pediatric Cardiac Surgery.* Mount Kisco, NY: Futura Publishing; 1989: 131–134.

40. Rizzoli G, Mazzucco A, Maizza F, Daliento L, Rubino M, Tursi V, Scalia D. Does Down syndrome affect prognosis of surgically managed atrioventricular canal defects? *J Thorac Cardiovasc Surg.* 1992;104: 945–953.

41. di Carlo DC, Marino B. Atrioventricular canal with Down syndrome or normal chromosome: distinct prognosis with surgical management? *J Thorac Cardiovasc Surg.* 1994;107(5):1368–1369.

CHAPTER 11

HEMODYNAMIC EVALUATION IN CHILDREN WITH DOWN SYNDROME AND CONGENITAL HEART DISEASE

Robert M. Freedom

PREVIOUS CHAPTERS IN THIS BOOK address the types and prevalence of congenital heart disease associated with Down syndrome (see also Chapters 7 and 10). For many years there has been the perception that patients with Down syndrome and congenital heart disease may be at higher risk for pulmonary vascular disease than patients with similar heart malformations but without Down syndrome (1–3) (see Chapters 8 and 13). The advocates for both sides of this discussion have been fairly persuasive in marshaling data to support their respective views. These particular issues are not repeated here; they have already been summarized (4). One can define a number of factors that may participate in the genesis of pulmonary vascular obstructive disease beyond the intrinsic character of the congenital heart malformation and the altitude at which the patient is living. These include the potential for chronic airway obstruction in the patient with Down syndrome. These children are known to have a small hypopharynx, and this is frequently compromised by the macroglossia and/or small oral cavity so common to the child with Down syndrome. These infants may somewhat underventilate with their hypotonia, thus developing nighttime hypercarbia and hypoxemia, again both stimuli for pulmonary vasoconstriction. The propensity for repeated upper and lower airway infections in these children may aggravate the potential for pulmonary vascular obstruction (4). However, the same concerns may be stated for the patient without Down syndrome. Thus, every patient with Down syndrome should have his or her history explored in terms of airway obstruction: nighttime snoring, sleep apnea, and so forth. An ear–nose–throat consultation is always an important consideration and adjunct in these patients.

THE OBLIGATORY LEFT-TO-RIGHT SHUNT

For the infant with Down syndrome and a biventricular heart being considered for complete repair of a cardiac malformation, what specific issues must be addressed? In some patients, despite clear-cut evidence of pulmonary hypertension, there will exist a clinically large left-to-right shunt. The question of operability on the basis of hemodynamics is not raised. In other patients the presence of an obligatory left-to-right shunt may confound this issue, and even at cardiac catheterization the calculated pulmonary vascular resistance and pulmonary arteriolar resistance may suggest operability when in fact there is advanced pulmonary vascular obstruction. The classic obligatory left-to-right shunt is seen in the patient with a complete form of atrioventricular septal defect (atrioventricular canal) and left atrioventricular valve regurgitation. The regurgitation is from left ventricle to right atrium, thus providing an obligatory left-to-right shunt that is independent of pulmonary vascular resistance. The recognition of an obligatory left-to-right shunt is important to the consideration of operability in these patients, and because hemodynamics may not provide definition the final arbiter may well be a lung biopsy. Indicator dye dilution techniques are not applicable to these patients because the atrioventricular valve regurgitation may distort the slope of the curve.

THE OBLIGATORY RIGHT-TO-LEFT SHUNT

It has been stated all too frequently that clinical cyanosis and hypoxemia in the patient whose underlying heart condition usually promotes a left-to-right shunt and pulmonary artery hypertension must have inoperable pulmonary vascular obstruction. However, there are a number of conditions that can promote an obligatory right-to-left shunt (5–7). These conditions are not specific to the patient with Down syndrome, but clearly these anomalies must be considered in any patient who is being excluded from surgical consideration. In the patient with a complete form of atrioventricular septal defect, a misaligned atrial septum producing a so-called double-outlet right atrium results in an obligatory right-to-left shunt (5–9). Similarly, connection of a left superior vena cava to the left atrium promotes hypoxemia and cyanosis. One must be cognizant of those diverse conditions causing an obligatory right-to-left shunt in the assessment of operability of these patients.

ASSESSMENT OF PULMONARY VASCULAR REACTIVITY IN THE CARDIAC CATHETERIZATION LABORATORY

It has been suggested elsewhere that patients with chronic airway disease should be studied while intubated and ventilated, thus obviating the adverse effects of chronic airway obstruction on the hemodynamics of these patients (4,10). Similarly, these patients should be studied in room air and in 100% inspired oxygen concentration. The calculations of pulmonary vascular resistance and pulmonary arteriolar resistance should be obtained with the patient in room air with measured oxygen consumption. Calculations should take into consideration dissolved oxygen. For those patients with large interventricular defects either in isolation or as part of an atrioventricular septal defect, pulmonary arterial pressures will reflect systemic pressures. The change in response to inspired oxygen rarely shows a striking diminution in PAp because this would necessitate a decline in systemic arterial pressure. Rather, a positive response to inspired oxygen shows a dramatic increase in Qp/Qs (pulmonary to systemic blood ratio and a fall in calculated pulmonary vascular resistance).

Some patients will have a large patent arterial duct complicating a smaller ventricular septal defect with or without an atrial septal defect. In the assessment of the pulmonary vascular bed, it may be important to study the hemodynamics of those particular patients with the arterial duct temporarily occluded with a balloon catheter. As a general guideline, these patients should be studied with classic oximetry as well as forward green dye curves. These curves will be very sensitive to detect right-to-left shunting. These curves can be performed in room air and, if there is evidence of right-to-left shunting, they can be repeated with the patients in increased ambient oxygen. The forward dye curves can be performed with injection of the green dye initially in the superior vena cava with sampling in the ascending aorta and then in the right ventricle with sampling in the aorta.

DOWN SYNDROME AND THE FONTAN PROCEDURE

A number of patients with Down syndrome will not be candidates for a biventricular repair because of ventricular hypoplasia. Although these patients may satisfy the static criteria for Fontan's operation or any of the many modifications, concerns about nighttime apnea and chronic nighttime hypoxemia and hypercarbia must be thoroughly evaluated, including a sleep study if necessary (10,11). Impedance to pulmonary blood flow by chronic though intermittent airway obstruction must be avoided.

REFERENCES

1. Chi TPL, Krovetz LJ. The pulmonary vascular bed in children with Down syndrome. *J Pediatr.* 1975;86:533–538.
2. Frescura C, Thiene G, Franceschini E, Talenti E, Mazzucco A. Pulmonary vascular disease in infants with complete atrioventricular septal defect. *Int J Cardiol.* 1987;15:91–100.
3. Rosengart RM. Pulmonary vascular involvement in Down syndrome. *J Pediatr.* 1976;88:161.
4. Freedom RM, Benson LN, Olley PM, Rowe RD. The natural history of the complete atrioventricular canal defect: an analysis of selected genetic, hemodynamic, and morphological variables. In: Gallucci V, Bini RM, Thiene G, eds. *Selected Topics in Cardiac Surgery.* Bologna: Patron Editore; 1980:45–72.
5. Corwin RD, Singh AK, Karlson KE. Double-outlet right atrium: a rare endocardial cushion defect. *Am Heart J.* 1983;106:1156–1157.
6. Alivizatos P, Anderson RH, Macarteney FJ, Zuberbuhler JR, Stark J. Atrioventricular septal defect with balanced ventricles and malaligned atrial septum: double-outlet right atrium. *J Thorac Cardiovasc Surg* 1985;89:295–297.
7. Ahmadi A, Mocellin R, Spillner G, Gildein HP. Atrioventricular septal defect with double-outlet right atrium. *Pediatr Cardiol.* 1989;10:170–173.
8. Soudon P, Stijns M, Tremouroux-Wattiez M, Vliers A. Precocity of pulmonary vascular obstruction in Down's syndrome. *Eur J Cardiol.* 1975;2:473–476.
9. Freedom RM, Benson LN. Anomalies of systemic venous connections, persistence of the right venous valve and silent cardiovascular causes of cyanosis. In: Freedom RM, Benson LN, Smallhorn JF, eds. *Neonatal Heart Disease.* London: Springer-Verlag; 1992:485–495.
10. Kasian GF, Duncan WJ, Tyrrell MJ, Oman-Ganes LA. Elective orotracheal intubation to diagnose sleep apnea syndrome in children with Down's syndrome and ventricular septal defect. *Can J Cardiol.* 1987; 3(1):2–5.
11. Choussat A, Fontan F, Besse P, Vallot F, Chauve A, Bricaud H. Selection criteria for Fontan's procedure. In: Anderson RH, Shinebourne EA, eds. *Paediatric Cardiology: 1977.* Edinburgh: Churchill Livingstone; 1978:559–566.

—————— CHAPTER *12*——————
ACCESS TO CARDIAC CARE FOR CHILDREN WITH DOWN SYNDROME

Edward B. Clark

CHILDREN WITH DOWN SYNDROME HAVE a 50% risk of developing congenital cardiovascular malformations compared with a 0.3% risk for infants who are chromosomally normal. In the Baltimore–Washington Infant Study, children with Down syndrome accounted for nearly 10% of all children identified with a congenital cardiovascular malformation (1).

For infants with Down syndrome, an aggressive approach to diagnosis and management is required because of the high frequency of severe congenital cardiovascular defects, the risk of rapid onset of irreversible pulmonary vascular damage, and the difficulty of diagnosis in some infants. Children with Down syndrome usually have severe heart defects including complete atrioventricular canal, ventricular septal defect, partial atrioventricular canal, atrial septal defect, tetralogy of Fallot, and patent ductus arteriosus. Complete atrioventricular canal defects account for about 60% of all cardiac defects, and all except tetralogy of Fallot have the potential to cause increased pulmonary blood flow and high pulmonary artery pressure.

It is essential that children with Down syndrome and congenital heart defects be recognized early in life in order to have the best opportunities for medical and surgical management (2). Those cardiac defects with increased pulmonary blood pressure and increased pulmonary blood flow have great potential for rapidly developing irreversible pulmonary vascular disease. These factors increase the stress–strain relationship in the pulmonary arterioles and rapidly lead to irreversible damage to the pulmonary vascular bed.

The pulmonary arterioles respond to chronic irritation by a staged response of medial hypertrophy and intimal proliferation. Although this response is not permanent in chromosomally normal children until about 2 years of age, children with Down syndrome have fixed vascular changes by 6–9 months. The reasons for this rapid development of pulmonary vascular damage are unclear, but contributing factors likely include upper airway obstruction, hypoxemia, hypercarbia, and intrinsic abnormalities of the pulmonary vascular bed (see Chapter 5).

DIAGNOSIS

The clinical recognition of heart defects in infants with Down syndrome may be enigmatic (3). Cardiac murmurs may be short or absent in infants with complete atrioventricular canal. Pulmonary artery hypertension may be apparent only as an increase in the intensity of the pulmonary component of the second heart sound. Infants with Down syndrome are difficult to examine because they often have rhonchus (i.e., airway noise from upper airway obstruction and persistent tachypnea). Some infants may not even have signs or symptoms of congestive heart failure because pulmonary vascular resistance remains high.

All infants with Down syndrome, including those without cardiac murmurs, must be examined for the possibility of congenital cardiovascular malformation. An initial evaluation should be performed at birth, including an electrocardiogram to search for abnormal counterclockwise superior loop on the frontal plane. It is essential, however, that the screening electrocardiogram be interpreted by a physician experienced in infant electrocardiography. In many communities, all infants with Down syndrome are referred for evaluation to a pediatric cardiologist. In communities where pediatric cardiology services are not readily available, infants without obvious evidence of cardiovascular disease should have a second electrocardiogram performed at 2 months of age. Infants with any abnormality on the electrocardiogram including a counterclockwise superior axis and/or right ventricular hypertrophy require further evaluation by a pediatric cardiologist. The pediatric cardiologist's evaluation should include a clinical assessment of the second heart sound, an electrocardiogram to search for abnormal frontal plane axis associated with atrioventricular canal defects or patterns of ventricular mass increase, a chest x-ray to evaluate cardiac size and pulmonary blood flow, and an echocardiogram to assess the atrioventricular valves and septa of the atria and ventricles. For some infants, cardiac catheterization may be necessary for complete delineation of cardiovascular abnormalities.

Whereas most severe congenital cardiac defects will be identified early, mild defects may require follow-up over an expanded period for definition. However, any congenital cardiovascular malformation that places the infant at risk for pulmonary artery hypertension must be identified before the baby is 4–6 months of age to permit planning for future care.

Historically, there have been barriers to care and management of congenital cardiovascular defects in infants with Down syndrome. Although this has been experienced by both parents and professionals for decades, attention was first drawn to the inequality of care in a study by Sondheimer and colleagues (4). They hypothesized that, despite the known high prevalence of congenital heart disease in Down syndrome, some children with Down syndrome were not being referred for pediatric cardiac evaluation at an early age. Of 36 children with complete atrioventricular canal, 28 had trisomy 21 and 8 had normal karyotype. All 8 chromosomally normal children with complete atrioventricular canal were evaluated before 1 year of age. Among the 28 children with Down syndrome, 18 were referred prior to 1 year of age and 17 of the 18 children were operable. Of the 10 children with Down syndrome initially seen when they were older than 1 year, only 5 were operable. Because the surgical management of a complete atrioventricular canal is aimed at avoiding pulmonary vascular disease and premature death, the late referral of this group of children with Down syndrome adversely affected the children's outcomes. Late referral could be avoided by early diagnosis and treatment.

SURGICAL TREATMENT

Another reason for the delay in the referral of children with Down syndrome has been a perception that they are at increased risk for operative treatment. In order to establish historical understanding, we analyzed 60 children with Down syndrome who were treated surgically between 1953 and 1975 at the Johns Hopkins Hospital (5). The overall mortality in these 60 patients was 30%, proportionately higher than that for more complex cardiac defects. In addition, we found that there was a marked reduction in the number and duration of hospitalizations in children surviving surgical repair from 3.0 admissions per patient to 0.6 admission per patient. Twenty-seven of the 47 children with Down syndrome surviving surgery had no subsequent hospitalizations. A reduction of hospitalizations sharply decreases costs to parents, the community, and the health care system in general.

An alternative view was given by Bull and colleagues, who presented the experience of Brompton Hospital from 1970 to 1975 (6). These pediatric cardiologists sought to establish a protocol for treatment of children with atrioventricular canal defects based on the presence or absence of Down syndrome. They found that all patients with Down syndrome had an 80% survival at 10–15 years and that surgical mortality was 20%. They suggested that parents be counseled as follows: Unless a surgical unit can offer very exceptional surgical results, survival through childhood is better with medical treatment. Although surgery offers the only chance for avoiding pulmonary vascular obstructive disease, there is an initial mortality of 30% and many survivors may have residual cardiovascular defects that will shorten their lives.

Bull and coworkers (6) found that decisions with regard to cardiac surgery correlated with the child's chromosomal state. Many parents of children with Down syndrome chose medical management, which often led to pulmonary vascular obstructive disease. Those with chromosomally normal children chose surgery. This finding is contrary to the usual patterns of care in the United States, in which all children, irrespective of their developmental disabilities, are afforded the same level of care.

There was a spirited response to the Bull et al. study (7). Most felt that surgery should be offered to all children with atrioventricular canal defect irrespective of any association with Down syndrome, provided that there is no surgical contraindication. Successful surgery results in an increasing cohort of adults with Down syndrome who will require long-term care. However, their care—whether at home with their families or in a custodial situation—will likely be easier and less expensive if the additional chronic complications of pulmonary vascular obstructive disease, cyanosis, and polycythemia can be avoided. In addition to longer survival, there should be improved health, which in turn reduces long-term medical costs.

Schneider and co-workers assessed the 1-year status of infants enrolled in the population-based Baltimore–Washington Infant Study from 1981 to 1986 (8). They compared the age at diagnosis, surgery, and survival of 166 infants with Down syndrome to 540 normal infants who had the same cardiac diagnosis and no chromosomal or extracardiac anomalies. By 26 weeks of age, 90% of infants with Down syndrome and normal infants with isolated cardiovascular malformation had been referred for cardiac diagnosis. Earlier diagnosis was made in infants with Down syndrome during the first 13 weeks of life compared to the chromosomally normal group.

The infants with Down syndrome were more likely to have undergone surgery before a year of age than those who were chromosomally normal. This probably reflects the aggressive management of children with excess pulmonary blood flow and pulmonary hypertension to avoid pulmonary vascular obstructive disease. The mortality at 1 year of age in surgically treated infants was similar in both groups. There was no difference in medical mortality at 1 year of age between infants with Down syndrome and those with isolated cardiac malformations. Thus, in a large metropolitan area there were no differences in the diagnosis and management of these groups of patients (8).

HEALTH INSURANCE

Another variable of health care delivery in the United States is the availability of health insurance. Unlike nearly all other industrialized nations, the United States does not provide universal assurance of health care for all citizens. We recently reviewed the database constructed of all patients seen at the pediatric cardiology division of the University of Rochester. We tabulated age, gender, diagnosis, severity of defect, and health insurance status for 5,448 patients seen from October 1987 to April 1991 (9). Of a cohort of 97 children with Down syndrome, 34% received state medical assistance, 29% belonged to a health maintenance organization, and 24% subscribed to fee-for-service plans like Blue Cross and Blue Shield or another commercial insurance. Among 25 young adults over the age of 21, 72% were covered by state insurance or Medicaid, 12% were covered by a health maintenance organization, and 16% subscribed to a fee-for-service plan. None were uninsured. This is in comparison to the chromosomally normal population in which nearly 50% of those over the age of 21 were uninsured or underinsured. All children with Down syndrome are eligible for health care benefits from the Social Security Administration and from state medical assistance programs.

Access to medical care for infants with Down syndrome depends on early and accurate diagnosis to preclude the development of fixed pulmonary vascular disease, surgical outcomes similar to that of chromosomally normal children with the same defect, and health insurance to cover the expense of medical and surgical treatment. In the long term, this appears to be a wise investment of medical and surgical resources. Aggressive medical and surgical care increases the likelihood that these children are likely to live longer than they would have in the era prior to surgical repair and decreases cumulative costs to families and society.

REFERENCES

1. Ferencz C, Correa-Villasenor A. Epidemiology of cardiovascular malformations: the state of the art. *Cardiol Young.* 1991;1:264–284.
2. Clark EB. Congenital cardiovascular defects in infants with Down syndrome. *Pediatr Rev.* 1989;11:99–100.
3. Tubman TRJ, Shields MD, Craig BG, Mulholland HC, Nevin NC. Congenital heart disease in Down's syndrome: two year prospective early screening study. *BMJ.* 1991;302:1425–1427.
4. Sondheimer HM, Byrum CJ, Blackman MS. Unequal cardiac care for children with Down syndrome. *Am J Dis Child.* 1985;139:68–70.
5. Katlic MR, Clark EB, Neill CA, Haller JA. Surgical management of congenital heart disease in Down's syndrome. *J Thorac Cardiovasc Surg.* 1977;74:204–209.
6. Bull C, Rigby ML, Shinebourne EA. Should management of complete atrioventricular canal defect be influenced by coexistent Down syndrome? *Lancet.* 1985;1:1147–1149.
7. Wilson NJ, Gavalaki E, Newman CGH, Menahem S, Mee RBB. Letters concerning complete atrioventricular canal defect in presence of Down syndrome (letter). *Lancet.* 1985;1:834–835.
8. Schneider DS, Zahka KG, Clark EB, Neill CA. Patterns of cardiac care in infants with Down syndrome. *Am J Dis Child.* 1989;143:363–365.
9. Truesdell SC, Clark EB. Health insurance status in a cohort of children and young adults with congenital cardiac diagnoses. *Circulation.* 1991; 84:II-386.

—————CHAPTER *13*—————

SHOULD COEXISTING DOWN SYNDROME AFFECT THE INDICATION FOR SURGERY OF CONGENITAL HEART DISEASE?

Duccio di Carlo

IN WESTERN SOCIETY, THE QUESTION of whether an infant with mental retardation should be offered surgical treatment of a correctable congenital heart defect is no longer debated. The quality of cardiac care for patients with Down syndrome is considered to be the same as that enjoyed by subjects who do not have Down syndrome (1–3). It is the general philosophy today that cardiac surgery be offered to persons with Down syndrome and to those with other chromosomal or nonchromosomal disorders that are known to result in mental retardation and shortened life expectancy. What is debated (4–8) is whether a similar or even better survival can be achieved in patients with Down syndrome without surgical treatment of coexisting congenital heart defects. This chapter reviews the existing information relative to indications for surgery of congenital heart defects in infants with Down syndrome.

COMPLETE ATRIOVENTRICULAR CANAL

The majority of subjects with complete atrioventricular canal have coexisting Down syndrome, whereas the opposite is true for the partial form of atrioventricular canal (9).

Preoperative Status

The repair of complete atrioventricular canal is a complex operation that must be performed early in life in order to prevent the occurrence of pulmonary vascular obstructive disease secondary to high pulmonary blood flow (10) (see Chapter 8). It has been stated that this complication rarely occurs before 1 year of life (10). In recent years, however, considerable evidence has accumulated regarding the accelerated development of pulmonary vascular obstructive disease in infants with Down syndrome and complete atrioventricular canal (10–16). This may in part be the consequence of extracardiac problems specific to patients with trisomy 21, such as upper airway obstruction (16–19), pulmonary hypoplasia (20), and/or immunologic deficiency (21). In addition, postoperative studies have demonstrated that infants with Down syndrome who survive the repair of complete atrioventricular canal tend to have higher pulmonary artery pressure and pulmonary resistance than patients who do not have Down syndrome (22). Initial stages of pulmonary vascular obstructive disease are suspected to be implicated in early postoperative death after apparently technically satisfactory operations (10). Similarly, the event of late death of patients with Down syndrome has often been attributed to evolving, irreversible pulmonary vascular obstructive disease.

Cardiac Anatomy

Recent studies have shown that the anatomic arrangement of complete atrioventricular canal in patients with Down syndrome is largely constant. Anomalies of the left atrioventricular valve apparatus, subaortic stenosis, and hypoplastic left ventricle (factors all known to increase the immediate risk of surgical repair) are rare (9,23–25). Their prevalence is, conversely, much higher in patients with normal genotype (23) (see Chapters 7 and 10).

Surgical Results

In the past, the immediate mortality of complete repair has been high (26–30), but results have improved greatly in recent years. Data relative to the experience acquired since the early 1980s in many centers throughout the world represent a mortality rate of 10% or less (8,31–38). An interesting observation is the lower mortality of children with Down syndrome in comparison with subjects who do not have Down syndrome. This phenomenon is usually attributed to the "simpler" anatomy in persons with trisomy 21 (31,39,40). The prevalence of reoperation because of left atrioventricular valve dysfunction is also lower in patients with Down syndrome. Williams and colleagues (32) reported that replacement of atrioventricular valve was required during or subsequent to repair of atrioventricular canal in 6 (81%) of 74 children with Down syndrome and 4 (17.4%) of 23 children without Down syndrome (41–43). When the presence of Down syndrome appeared to increase the immediate surgical risk, a confounding effect of other factors such as pulmonary and infective complications was often found at closer examination of the data by multivariate analysis (21,26).

The conclusion reached in many published papers is that coexisting Down syndrome either has no adverse effect on immediate survival at repair of complete atrioventricular canal or has a favorable effect (25,32,40). Data pointing to the opposite conclusion are most likely the result of the early occurrence of pulmonary vascular obstructive disease and untimely referral for surgery (1).

Medical versus Surgical Treatment

In a recent paper (44), Samanek pointed out that in a historical series 59 of 60 unoperated patients with Down syndrome and complete atrioventricular canal died before reaching their first birthday. Similar data (96% mortality at 5-year follow-up) had been published by Berger and colleagues (27) in 1979 based on a review of autopsy cases.

Conversely, Bull and co-workers (4) quoted a much better survival of patients with Down syndrome and complete atrioventricular canal with medical treatment alone. An 80% actuarial survival at 10 years was reported by these authors. These data were difficult to match by surgical treatment at the time of writing. Admittedly, all survivors had evolving pulmonary vascular obstructive disease, which was expected to cause their death during the third decade of life. Given the reduced life expectancy of persons with Down syndrome, this time span was not judged unacceptable (4).

A series of criticisms have been raised (4,5):

1. In the series originally described, the actuarial curve indicated an 80% survival at 10 years but less than 50% of the initial patients entered in fifth year of follow-up (6). Moreover, the entering point was indicated as birth although it should have been time of referral (8). The authors state in fact that no indication for surgery seems reasonable beyond 1 year of life (5). This may be true for patients with Down syndrome because of early devel-

opment of pulmonary vascular obstructive disease. What is also implicit in Bull and co-workers' data is that younger patients were referred for surgery by virtue of their more severe clinical condition as they would likely have died with medical treatment alone. Consequently, mortality, if any, was somehow "shifted" to the surgical series.

2. An institutional bias of referral for medical treatment of complete atrioventricular canal in patients with Down syndrome probably does occur in the authors' clinical practice (6).

3. When reviewing the unfavorable results of complete atrioventricular canal surgery, Bull and colleagues failed to appreciate the different results in each series between subjects with Down syndrome and those without Down syndrome. As we have previously seen, these findings are fairly constant in the recent literature and can in fact be extrapolated from the data produced by the authors in their original paper (6).

4. The results of cardiac surgery in children with Down syndrome have greatly improved since the time of the original Bull et al. report. Similar or even better actuarial survival can be predicted with surgery and the vast majority of survivors are expected to be free of cardiovascular symptoms. The burden for families and society of a cyanotic individual with overt signs of right heart failure should not be underestimated. Reoperation hazard still is not zero but, as mentioned, it seems usually to concern patients with normal karyotype (31,41–43).

We believe, therefore, that surgical treatment of complete atrioventricular canal should not be denied to individuals because they have Down syndrome. Early referral (within 6 months of age) and intervention should be pursued. A positive effect on long-term survival and well-being of these persons can be anticipated. Survival proportion should then approach that of persons with Down syndrome without a cardiac defect (45).

OTHER CARDIOVASCULAR ANOMALIES

Fewer data are available regarding the treatment of congenital heart defects other than complete atrioventricular canal in patients with Down syndrome.

Ventricular Septal Defect

A specific anatomic characteristic with regard to ventricular septal defect has been noted in children with Down syndrome (46,47) (see Chapters 7 and 10). In a paper concerning the repair of ventricular septal defects in patients with normal karyotype and in patients with Down syndrome, a propensity for pulmonary complications was described (48). Preoperatively, a higher pulmonary artery pressure was found on average in the group of children with Down syndrome than in subjects who do not have Down syndrome. This finding did not correlate with the age at time of referral. As for patients with Down syndrome and complete atrioventricular canal, accelerated pulmonary vascular obstructive disease could be a major determinant of mortality and morbidity at the time of the repair of the ventricular septal defect. Our clinical experience is similar to that of others inasmuch as an increased prevalence of pulmonary complications in patients with Down syndrome was noted.

Tetralogy of Fallot

Very few reports deal with the risk of repair of patients with tetralogy of Fallot and Down syndrome. In a small series of operations performed between 1953 and 1975 the mortality was 60% (49). The authors stated correctly that improvements of results with refined techniques would also positively affect children with Down syndrome.

A recent paper with a large series from two leading institutions (50) reported a higher surgical mortality in patients with Down syndrome in comparison with those who do not have Down syndrome. However, this influence was no longer evident once the confounding effect of associated complete atrioventricular canal was eliminated.

In our experience, patients with Down syndrome and tetralogy of Fallot frequently present severe forms of right ventricular outflow tract obstruction and require transannular patching; this may explain the possibly increased surgical risk in this population. Early surgical repair to neutralize the negative effects of transannular patching (50) may be advantageous in children with Down syndrome.

Fontan Operation

To our knowledge, the Fontan operation (or a modification) has never been performed in patients with Down syndrome. As suggested elsewhere in this book (see Chapter 11), this operation could be performed provided intensive preoperative evaluation of the candidate was conducted to rule out constant or nocturnal hypercarbia by chronic airway obstruction or sleep apnea. Short of such an ideal surgical candidate, the opportunity to treat individuals with Down syndrome with the Fontan operation should be extremely rare. Since the prevalence of hypoplastic right/left ventricle is low, indication for the Fontan operation will be exceptional (see Chapters 7 and 10). We successfully performed a bidirectional cavopulmonary shunt following pulmonary artery banding in a patient with Down syndrome, complete atrioventricular canal, and unbalanced ventricles. At present, this patient is not a candidate for further interventions.

HEART/LUNG TRANSPLANTATION

A unique case of lung transplantation and repair of intracardiac defects in a patient with Down syndrome has recently been described (51). Although in this case an approach of considerable interest was chosen, the shortage of organs may preclude its widespread acceptance.

CONCLUSIONS

There are no obvious medical or ethical reasons for treating persons with Down syndrome differently from chromosomally normal patients. It is hard to imagine that a patient with restricted pulmonary blood flow, either from birth or because of early occurring pulmonary vascular obstructive disease, should be happier or more self-sufficient than a person without cardiac disabilities. The existing data nevertheless indicate that earlier treatment of cardiac defects with pulmonary hypertension is mandatory in order to significantly affect the life expectancy of individuals with Down syndrome. Postoperative care should be tailored to match the multiple problems of Down syndrome. At present, the only contraindicated type of surgery is represented by the Fontan operation or, at least, by its indiscriminate use.

REFERENCES

1. Schneider DS, Zahka KG, Clark EB, Neill CA. Patterns of cardiac care in infants with Down syndrome. *Am J Dis Child.* 1989;143:363–365.
2. Sondheimer HM, Byrum CJ, Blackman MS. Unequal cardiac care for children with Down's syndrome. *Am J Dis Child.* 1985;139:68–70.
3. Silberbach M, Shumaker D, Menashe V, Cobanoglu A, Morris C. Predicting hospital charge and length of stay for congenital heart disease surgery. *Am J Cardiol.* 1993;72:958–963.
4. Bull C, Rigby M, Shinebourne EA. Should management of complete atrioventricular canal defect be influenced by coexistent Down's syndrome? *Lancet.* 1985;1:1147–1149.
5. Shinebourne E, Carvalho J, Rigby M. Atrioventricular septal defect with Down's syndrome—late results of non-surgical management. *Cardiol Young.* 1993;3(1):47.
6. Wilson NJ, Gavalaki E, Newman CGH. Complete atrioventricular canal defect in presence of Down syndrome. *Lancet.* 1985;2:834.
7. Menahem S, Mee RBB. Complete atrioventricular canal defect in presence of Down syndrome. *Lancet.* 1985;2:834–835.

8. Kirklin JW, Blackstone EH, Bargeron LM, Pacifico AD, Kirklin JK. The repair of atrioventricular septal defects in infancy. *Int J Cardiol.* 1986;13:333–351.

9. Marino B, Vairo U, Corno A, et al. Atrioventricular canal in Down syndrome: prevalence of associated cardiac malformations compared with patients without Down syndrome. *Am J Dis Child.* 1990;144: 1120–1122.

10. Soudon P, Stijns M, Tremouroux-Wattiez M, Vliers A. Precocity of pulmonary vascular obstruction in Down's syndrome. *Eur J Cardiol.* 1975;2/4:473–476.

11. Chi TL, Krovets JL. The pulmonary vascular bed in children with Down syndrome. *J Pediatr.* 1975;86:533–538.

12. Haworth SG. Pulmonary vascular bed in children with complete atrioventricular septal defect: relation between structural and hemodynamic abnormalities. *Am J Cardiol.* 1986;57:833–839.

13. Frescura C, Thiene G, Franceschini E, Talenti E, Mazzucco A. Pulmonary vascular disease in infants with complete atrioventricular septal defects. *Int J Cardiol.* 1987;15:91–100.

14. Clapp S, Perry BP, Farooki ZQ, et al. Down's syndrome, complete atrioventricular canal and pulmonary vascular obstructive disease. *J Thorac Cardiovasc Surg.* 1990;100:115–121.

15. Yamaki S, Yasui H, Kado H, et al. Pulmonary vascular disease and operative indications in complete atrioventricular canal defect in early infancy. *J Thorac Cardiovasc Surg.* 1993;106:398–405.

16. Clark RW, Schmidt HS, Schuller DE. Sleep-induced ventilatory dysfunction in Down's syndrome. *Arch Intern Med.* 1980;140:45–50.

17. Rowland TW, Nordstrom LG, Bean MS, Burkhardt H. Chronic upper airway obstruction and pulmonary hypertension in Down's syndrome. *Am J Dis Child.* 1981;135:1050–1052.

18. Loughlin GM, Wynne JW, Victorica BE. Sleep apnea as a possible cause of pulmonary hypertension in Down syndrome. *J Pediatr.* 1981; 98:435–437.

19. Kobel M, Creighton RE, Steward DJ. Anaesthetic consideration in Down's syndrome: experience with 100 patients and review of the literature. *Can Anaesth Soc J.* 1982;29:593–599.

20. Cooney TP, Thurlbeck WM. Pulmonary hypoplasia in Down's syndrome. *N Engl J Med.* 1982;307:1170–1173.

21. Spina CA, Smith D, Korn E, Fahey JL, Grossman HJ. Altered cellular immune functions in patients with Downs syndrome. *Am J Dis Child.* 1981;135:251–255.

22. Morris CD, Magilke D, Reller M. Down's syndrome affects results of surgical correction of complete atrioventricular canal. *Pediatr Cardiol.* 1992;13:80–84.

23. De Biase L, Di Ciommo V, Ballerini L, Bevilacqua M, Marcelletti C, Marino B. Prevalence of left-sided obstructive lesions in patients with atrioventricular canal without Down's syndrome. *J Thorac Cardiovasc Surg.* 1986;91:467–469.

24. Marino B. Atrioventricular septal defect: anatomic characteristics in patients with and without Down's syndrome. *Cardiol Young.* 1992;2: 308–310.

25. Di Carlo D, Marino B. Atrioventricular canal with Down's syndrome or normal chromosomes; distinct prognosis with surgical management? *J Thorac Cardiovasc Surg.* 1994;107(5):1368–1369.
26. Cooper DKC, de Leval MR, Stark J. Results of surgical correction of persistent atrioventricular canal. *J Thorac Cardiovasc Surg.* 1979;79: 11–15.
27. Berger TJ, Blackstone EH, Kirklin JW, Bargeron LM Jr, Hazelrig JB, Turner ME Jr. Survival and probability of cure without and with operation in complete atrioventricular canal. *Ann Thorac Surg.* 1979;27: 104–111.
28. Chin AJ, Keane JF, Norwood WI, Castaneda AR. Repair of complete common atrioventricular canal in infancy. *J Thorac Cardiovasc Surg.* 1982;84:437–445.
29. Studer M, Blackstone EH, Kirklin JW, et al. Determinants of early and late results of repair of atrioventricular septal (canal) defects. *J Thorac Cardiovasc Surg.* 1982;84:523–542.
30. Rizzoli G, Mazzucco A, Maizza F, et al. Does Down syndrome affect prognosis of surgically managed atrioventricular canal defects? *J Thorac Cardiovasc Surg.* 1992;104:945–953.
31. McGrath LB, Gonzalez-Lavin L. Actuarial survival, freedom from reoperation and other events after repair of atrioventricular septal defects. *J Thorac Cardiovasc Surg.* 1987;94:582–590.
32. Williams WH, Perrella AM, Plauth WH Jr, Hatcher CR Jr, Guyton RA. Survival following repair of complete atrioventricular canal associated with Down's syndrome. In: Crupi G, Parenzan L, Anderson RH, eds. *Perspectives in Pediatric Cardiology.* Vol 2. Mount Kisco, NY: Futura Publishing; 1989:131–134.
33. Weintraub RG, Brawn WJ, Venables AW, Mee RBB. Two-patch repair of complete atrioventricular septal defect in the first year of life. *J Thorac Cardiovasc Surg.* 1990;99:320–326.
34. Lacour-Gayet F, Comas J, Bruniaux J, et al. Management of the left atrioventricular valve in 95 patients with atrioventricular septal defects and a common atrioventricular orifice. A ten year review. *Cardiol Young.* 1991;1:367–373.
35. Merrill WH, Hammon JW Jr, Bender HW Jr. Technique of repair of atrioventricular septal defect with common atrioventricular orifice. *Cardiol Young.* 1991;1:379–382.
36. Pozzi M, Remig J, Fimmers R, Urban AE. Atrioventricular septal defects: analysis of short- and medium-term results. *J Thorac Cardiovasc Surg.* 1991;101:138–142.
37. Hanley FL, Fenton KN, Jonas RA, et al. Surgical repair of complete atrioventricular canal defects in infancy. *J Thorac Cardiovasc Surg.* 1993;106:387–397.
38. Hashmat Ashraf M, Amin Z, Sharma R, Subramanian S. Atrioventricular canal defect: two-patch repair and tricuspidalization of the mitral valve. *Ann Thorac Surg.* 1993;55:347–351.
39. Barrat-Boyes BG. Atrioventricular canal defect: introduction. In: Crupi G, Parenzan L, Anderson RH, eds. *Perspectives in Pediatric Cardiology.* Vol 2. Mount Kisco, NY: Futura Publishing; 1989:73–80.
40. Vet TW, Ottenkamp J. Correction of atrioventricular septal defect: results influenced by Down syndrome? *Am J Dis Child.* 1989;143: 1361–1365.

41. Abbruzzese PA, Napoleone A, Bini M, Annecchino FP, Merlo M, Parenzan L. Late left atrioventricular valve insufficiency after repair of partial atrioventricular septal defects: anatomic and surgical determinants. *Ann Thorac Surg* 1990;49:111–114.
42. Marino B. Valve insufficiency after atrioventricular septal defect repair: differences between patients with and without Down's syndrome? *Ann Thorac Surg.* 1990;50:854.
43. Di Carlo D, Ballerini L, Tomasco B, Carotti A, Marcelletti C. E'definitiva la correzione del difetto settale atrioventricolare completo? *G Ital Cardiol.* 1992;22(2):7.
44. Samanek M. Prevalence at birth, natural risk and survival with atrioventricular septal defect. *Cardiol Young.* 1991;1:285–289.
45. Fabia J, Drollette M. Life tables up to age 10 for mongols with and without congenital heart defect. *J Ment Defic Res.* 1970;14:235–242.
46. Marino B, Papa M, Guccione P, Corno A, Marasini M, Calabró R. Ventricular septal defect in Down syndrome. Anatomic types and associated malformation. *Am J Dis Child* 1990;144:544–545.
47. Marino B, Corno A, Guccione P, Marcelletti C. Ventricular septal defect and Down's syndrome. *Lancet.* 1991;2:245–246.
48. Morray JP, Mac Gillivray R, Duker G. Increased perioperative risk following repair of congenital heart disease in Down's syndrome. *Anaesthesiology.* 1986;65:221–224.
49. Katlic MR, Clark EB, Neill C, Haller JA Jr. Surgical management of congenital heart disease in Down's syndrome. *J Thorac Cardiovasc Surg.* 1977;74:204–209.
50. Kirklin JW, Blakstone EH, Jonas RA, et al. Morphologic and surgical determinants of outcome events after repair of tetralogy of Fallot and pulmonary stenosis. *J Thorac Cardiovasc Surg.* 1992;103:706–723.
51. Bridges ND, Mallory GB Jr, Huddleston CB, Canter CE, Sweet SC, Spray TL. Lung transplantation in children and young adults with cardiovascular disease. *Ann Thorac Surg.* 1995;59:813–821.

————————— Chapter *14*—————————

SURGICAL INTERVENTION AND POSTOPERATIVE RESULTS IN PATIENTS WITH CONGENITAL HEART DISEASE AND DOWN SYNDROME

Hillel Laks and Jeffrey M. Pearl

T HE ASSOCIATION BETWEEN DOWN SYNDROME and congenital heart disease has long fascinated the medical community. Interest in this association has concentrated on a wide variety of areas including the specific defects and the particular features associated with those lesions. The pulmonary vasculature has been of great concern as early reports suggested an increased tendency for irreversible pulmonary vascular disease in patients with Down syndrome and atrioventricular canal (1). The various differences between patients with and without Down syndrome and congenital heart disease may influence the surgical approach and outcome.

The incidence of heart defects in children with Down syndrome ranges from 40% to 70% according to various series (2). The most common lesion associated with Down syndrome is atrioventricular canal. However, isolated ventricular septal defects or a ventricular septal defect with a secundum atrial septal defect is also common. Inlet ventricular septal defects seem to have an increased prevalence in patients with Down syndrome compared with predominantly perimembranous defects in patients with normal chromosomes. Furthermore, atrioventricular canal in children with Down syndrome usually occurs as an isolated cardiac defect with a lower prevalence of obstructive lesions of the right or left ventricle as compared with atrioventricular canal without Down syndrome (3,4). The occurrence of unbalanced atrioventricular canals is also uncommon in patients with Down syndrome. These differences influence both the surgical timing and the choice of operation for these patients.

The natural history of complete atrioventricular canal predicts only 54% survival to 6 months of age and 15% survival to 2 years of age without surgical intervention (5). The presence of Down syndrome has a negative effect on the natural history of atrioventricular canal (2). Late survival is also decreased in patients with Down syndrome undergoing surgical repair of atrioventricular canal compared to that in patients with normal karyotype (6,7).

These observations on long-term survival in patients with Down syndrome, in conjunction with initial reports of high operative mortality, raised an ethical question as to whether definitive repair was indicated (8). However, with improvement in operative techniques, early mortality for repair of atrioventricular canal has decreased to 5%–15% in most recent series (9–11). Furthermore, the presence of Down syndrome does not appear to affect the early mortality in most current series (2,10–12). Earlier operative intervention, improved surgical techniques, and better postoperative care are responsible for the improved results for patients with atrioventricular canal, both those with and those without Down syndrome. It is our opinion that barring significant associated anomalies, such as documented irreversible pulmonary hypertension (>10 Wood U/m^2), definitive repair should be offered to all patients with atrioventricular canal. The presence of Down syndrome is not "per se" a contraindication for surgery.

PULMONARY ARTERY BANDING

In early experiences with atrioventricular canal, when the mortality for complete repair was high, pulmonary artery banding was a popular approach to the infant with an atrioventricular canal and congestive heart failure. However, as results with complete repair in infancy have continued to improve, the indication for pulmonary artery banding has decreased (13–15). In general, pulmonary artery banding is reserved for 1) patients in congestive heart failure who are very small; 2) patients with sepsis; 3) patients with severe associated cardiac lesions, particularly left-sided obstructive lesions such as coarctation or a hypoplasic aortic arch; 4) patients with an unbalanced canal with a very small right or left ventricle; or 5) patients with significant noncardiac defects such as duodenal atresia. Concomitant coarctation repair or ductus arteriosus ligation can be successfully carried out at the time of pulmonary artery banding. When pulmonary artery banding is required, we have used an adjustable band that allows for control of pulmonary flow in the postoperative period. In our experience, achieving and maintaining the appropriate amount of pulmonary flow can be quite difficult. Pulmonary artery banding may fail to protect the pulmonary vascular bed, and bands may also migrate out of position causing stenosis and deformity of the branch pulmonary arteries if they are too distal or if distortion of the pulmonary valve is too proximal. Erosion of a pulmonary artery may also occur. Patients with severe congestive heart failure who have evidence of severe mitral regurgitation are not appropriately treated by banding but rather should undergo complete repair.

SURGICAL TIMING FOR CORRECTION

Atrioventricular Canal

Irreversible pulmonary vascular disease begins to occur by 6 months of age in patients with atrioventricular canal and may also be present in those with a large isolated ventricular septal defect (6). Subtle changes may be seen earlier, however, and experience has shown that even 3-month-old patients may have some degree of irreversibility (16). By 2 years of age patients with unprotected pulmonary vascular bed will have severe and irreversible pulmonary vascular disease that often precludes definitive repair.

Patients with Down syndrome and either an atrioventricular canal or an isolated ventricular septal defect are considered to have more advanced pulmonary vascular disease at a comparable age than patients without Down syndrome (1). However, clinical experience has brought into question the validity and significance of this finding with comparable surgical results in both groups (2,6,17,18). Perhaps, as suggested by Clapp and co-workers (1), a higher percentage of patients with Down syndrome develop irreversible pulmonary vascular disease and are not referred for surgery; thus, surgical series may be biased in favor of patients with Down syndrome. Regardless of the degree of preoperative fixed pulmonary vascular disease, patients with Down syndrome do have increased airway reactivity, which may precipitate acute increases in pulmonary vascular resistance in the postoperative period. Early repair also avoids the potential complications of pulmonary artery banding and ensures that no further damage to the pulmonary vascular bed will occur.

Although early surgical repair of atrioventricular canal lesions is favored and will prevent progression of pulmonary vascular disease, increased vasoreactivity is present in some young infants, which can complicate the postoperative course. For this reason, elective surgical repair is postponed until after 3 months of age unless symptoms occur. Most patients do not develop significant symptoms of congestive heart failure until after 3 months of age and hence most surgical repairs are performed at our institution between 3 and 6 months of age. Recent reports demonstrate a low mortality in patients 3–12 months old at the time of definitive repair (17,19–23). Results in infants less than 3 months old are also good, but the numbers are small. Surgical mortality is probably comparable between the ages of 3 and 12 months. We advocate definitive repair of complete atrioventricular canal defects by 6 months of age, and preferably between 3 and 6 months of age.

Ventricular Septal Defects

Children with Down syndrome and isolated ventricular septal defects tend to have larger defects than patients with normal chromosomes. Combined with an increased tendency toward irreversible pulmonary vascular disease, earlier operative intervention is indicated.

SURGICAL TECHNIQUE FOR CORRECTION

Determining the success of surgical repair of atrioventricular canal is based not only on the early mortality but on the reoperation rate as well. The early mortality for surgical repair of an atrioventricular canal has decreased since the 1980s as a result of improved methods of myocardial protection, better postoperative care, and improved understanding of operation indications including the selective use of pulmonary artery banding. The two main controversies regarding repair of complete atrioventricular canal include the method of closure of the interventricular and interatrial defects (i.e., single- vs. double-patch technique) and the treatment of the mitral valve as a bileaflet valve. The different approaches may influence the early mortality rate and outcome, especially if mitral insufficiency is present in the post-repair patient. Additionally, the surgical approach may influence the reoperation rate and hence the long-term survival rate.

Cardiopulmonary Bypass and Myocardial Protection

Following mean sternotomy the heart is exposed and a generous piece of pericardium excised (usually 4 × 5 cm). The pericardium is stretched on a piece of plastic, bathed in 0.6% gluteraldehyde for 2 minutes, and rinsed in saline. In patients with Down syndrome a submammary incision is not employed. Cardiopulmonary bypass is instituted with bicaval cannulation and the aorta is cross-clamped when the perfusate reaches 24°C. An initial dose of warm amino acid–enriched blood cardioplegia is given. Following arrest, the cardioplegia is cooled to 6°C and given for an additional 2 minutes. In infants weighing less than 6 kg, cardioplegia is delivered by hand with a syringe and infusion pressure monitored (40–40 mm Hg). In infants weighing more than 6 kg, cardioplegia is given via the cardioplegia line at a pressure of 80 mm Hg initially, then 60 mm Hg once arrest is achieved. The left ventricle is vented during cardioplegia administration via a DLP vent (DLP Inc., Grand Rapids, Michigan) placed via the right superior pulmonary vein. Cooling is continued to 22°C in infants weighing over 4 kg and to 20°C for those under 4 kg.

More recently, retrograde cardioplegia via the coronary sinus has also been used to further improve myocardial protection. Antegrade cardioplegia is given every 20 minutes for 2 minutes. Retrograde cardioplegia is given for 1–10 minutes following each antegrade dose. Warm glutamate- and aspartate-enriched blood cardioplegia is also given prior to release of the aortic cross-clamp.

Repair of the Mitral Component of the Atrioventricular Canal

The left atrioventricular valve may be treated either as a trileaflet or bileaflet valve. The particular approach used influences the incidence of postoperative atrioventricular valve regurgitation and the need for reoperation. We have adopted a protocol of routine suturing of the septal commissure (cleft), thus treating the valve as a bileaflet structure (Figure 1). Valve annuloplasty is also used liberally (Figure 2). Intraoperative assessment of the left atrioventricular valve is crucial in determining the need for annuloplasty and further valve repair. Postoperative mitral valve regurgitation is poorly tolerated and results in a high mortality unless prompt reoperation is undertaken. Following cleft suture, the valve is again tested; if it remains incompetent, commissural annuloplasty should be performed to eliminate any central leak resulting from annular dilatation or deficiency of valvar tissue. Annuloplasty is performed across the lateral commissures of the left atrioventricular valve which effectively reduces the valvar circumference without causing stenosis (Figure 3). A detailed description of our techniques of managing the left atrioventricular valve and the single-patch technique for atrioventricular canal repair was published previously (12).

Carpentier reported a low incidence of reoperation for residual mitral regurgitation when treating the valve as a trileaflet structure (24). Although Carpentier and others advocate a trileaflet approach

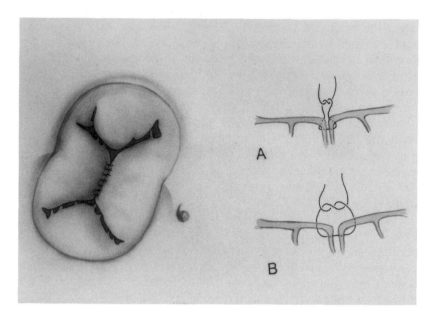

Figure 1.   Suture of the commissure with interrupted sutures with insets demonstrating correct **(A)** and incorrect **(B)** placement.

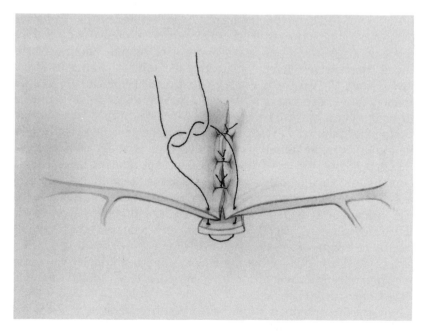

Figure 2.   Pericardial pledget to reinforce suture of the septal commissure.

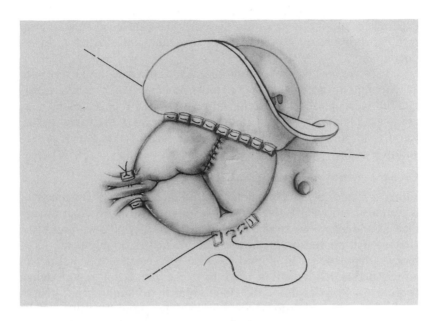

Figure 3. Annuloplasty with multiple pericardial pledgets at the lateral commissure.

(24,25), most surgeons have found the trileaflet approach to be associated with a higher prevalence of residual regurgitation and therefore prefer a bileaflet approach (11,18,26,27). Using a selective approach with cleft suturing only as indicated, McGrath and co-workers (18) reported reoperation for valve incompetence in 11 of 46 patients (24%). The 10-year actual rate of freedom from reoperation was only 68%. Many of these valves could not be repaired and most patients required valve replacement (18). Pozzi and co-workers (11) reported a 10.9% prevalence of reoperation for failure of atrioventricular valve repair at a mean of 7.2 months postoperatively. Actuarial rate of freedom from the need for reoperation was 84% at 80 months. Pozzi and co-workers switched to a bileaflet approach partway through their series due to dissatisfaction with the trileaflet approach (11).

We previously showed a significant decrease in mitral regurgitation on echocardiography and a low prevalence of reoperation (8%) with the bileaflet approach (12). In our series, postoperative echocardiography revealed no mitral valve insufficiency in 32%, mild mitral valve insufficiency in 52%, moderate mitral valve insufficiency in 15%, and severe mitral valve insufficiency in only 1% of patients. Preoperative echocardiographic data from this group of patients revealed 24% with moderate or severe atrioventricular valve regurgitation compared with only 12% postoperatively ($p = .03$). In our experience, routine cleft suture and the liberal use of annuloplasty resulted in improved mitral valve competence and a low rate of re-operation.

Valve replacement is rarely necessary either at initial repair or at reoperation. In our experience, most reoperations for valve regurgitation were the result of technical errors in the repair, usually separation of previously sutured clefts or malposition of the valvar tissue. Reoperation for left atrioventricular valve incompetence involves re-suturing of the cleft and valve annuloplasty.

Closure of the Atrioventricular Canal

Either a single- or double-patch technique can be used for repair of a complete atrioventricular canal. Although there is no clear advantage of one technique over the other (10,11,15,27,28), we prefer the single-patch approach (Figures 4 and 5). In the double-patch technique a synthetic patch is used to close the ventricular septal defect and a pericardial patch is used to close the atrial septal defect (Figure 6). Proponents of the double-patch technique argue that it results in less valvar distortion and less shortening of the valve leaflets than with the single-patch technique because the valve is not divided. However, valve division provides for better exposure of the ventricular septal defect and more precise ventricular septal defect closure.

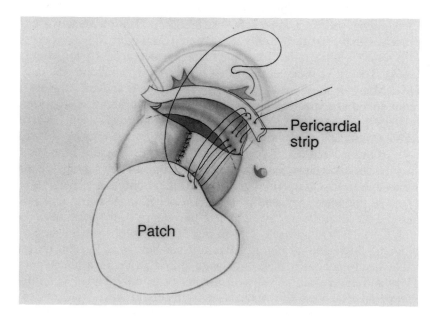

Figure 4. Suture of patch to ventricular septum with pericardial strip.

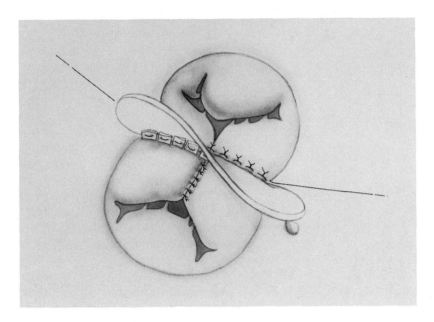

Figure 5. Completed attachment of valvar leaflets to the patch.

Therefore, a proposed advantage of the single-patch technique is a lower prevalence of residual shunting. In addition, pericardium alone can be used for the repair, thus avoiding the need for prosthetic material.

Closure of an Isolated Ventricular Septal Defect

Ventricular septal defects in patients with Down syndrome tend to be more posterior and larger (inlet ventricular septal defect) than in patients with normal karyotype, and early intervention is often required. The cordae of the tricuspid valve may require transection and re-attachment in order to expose and repair an inlet ventricular septal defect. Because of the position and larger size, there is an increased risk of injury to the conduction tissue when closing a ventricular septal defect in a patient with Down syndrome. However, the frequency of complete heart block remains low.

POSTOPERATIVE CARE

The purpose of postoperative care of patients with Down syndrome undergoing surgical repair of atrioventricular canal or an isolated ventricular septal defect is to prevent pulmonary hypertensive crises. Stimuli of pulmonary vasospasm such as hypoxia, hypercapnea, ac-

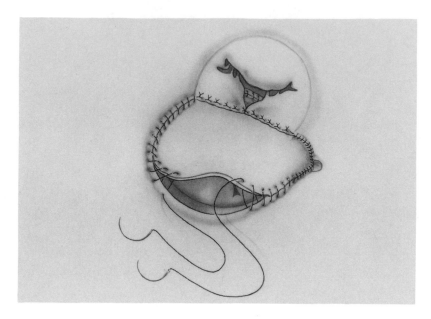

Figure 6. Closure of the atrial septal defect.

idosis, pain, and hypothermia must be avoided. In general, patients are sedated with fentanyl and paralyzed. Mechanical ventilation is maintained for 24–48 hours. Prostaglandin E_1 and nitroglycerin can be beneficial in lowering pulmonary vascular resistance. Cardiac output and blood pressure are supported with dopamine and dobutamine. Care must be taken to avoid the buildup of secretions in the tracheobronchial tree. In our experience, patients with Down syndrome have a tendency for increased pulmonary secretions. Policy in our intensive care units dictates that endotracheal suctioning be carried out with two nurses at the bedside. Hypoxia must be avoided during suctioning in these patients. Pulmonary hypertensive crises may also be triggered by suctioning. A plugged endotracheal tube must be considered in any patient who develops unexplained hypoxia or bradycardia.

SURGICAL RESULTS IN PATIENTS WITH DOWN SYNDROME AND CONGENITAL HEART DISEASE: UCLA EXPERIENCE

A total of 176 patients with a diagnosis of Down syndrome have undergone surgery for a congenital heart defect at the UCLA Medical Center from 1982 to March 1993. This series does not include patients referred to our institution who were not operated. Furthermore, the frequency of the various cardiac defects and their severity may be biased by referral patterns. Of the 176 patients, 119 (67%) had a primary diagnosis of atrioventricular canal; 114 of these were complete atrioventricular canals with five being unbalanced. Seven patients had an additional muscular ventricular septal defect, 25 had a secundum atrial septal defect, four had pulmonary stenosis or subpulmonic stenosis, five had associated tetralogy of Fallot, and one had left ventricular outflow tract obstruction. The mean age of the children was 18.5 months and the median age was 8 months. One hundred and eleven patients underwent complete surgical repair using a single-patch technique and treatment of the atrioventricular valve as a bileaflet structure. Fourteen patients had an additional ventricular septal defect closed and 25 had a secundum atrial septal defect or foramen ovale closed. The overall early mortality was 5.4% (6 of 111). In patients with atrioventricular canal repair alone with or without ductus arteriosus ligation, the early mortality was 4.0% (3 of 75). In the 14 patients who had undergone prior pulmonary artery banding, there were no early deaths.

An additional 24 patients underwent surgical repair for isolated ventricular septal defects and 26 patients for ventricular septal defect associated with a secundum atrial septal defect. Of the 56 ventricular septal defects in this series, 19 were inlet, 25 were perimembranous, 10 were muscular, and two were malaligned defects. Additional procedures included ligation of a ductus arteriosus in 16 patients. The early mortality in this group of patients was 4% (2 of 50). Other procedures included repair of tetralogy of Fallot in two patients, Glenn shunt in four, Rastelli procedure in one, and mitral and tricuspid valve repair in one patient.

Thirteen patients with complete atrioventricular canal underwent pulmonary artery banding combined with ductus arteriosus ligation in eight patients at a mean age of 4 months. There were no early deaths in this group. The overall early mortality for all operations in this group of 176 patients with Down syndrome was 5.1% (9 of 176). During the same time period we also evaluated 50 patients with atrioventricular canal who did not have Down syndrome. The frequency of left ventricular outflow obstruction or coarctation was 11% and the frequency of right ventricular outflow tract obstruction of tetralogy of Fallot was 17%. Thirty-eight had complete atrioventricular canal defect and underwent definitive repair. Eight patients had undergone previous pulmonary artery banding. The operative mortality of this group of children was 11.8%. Of interest is the prevalence of associated obstructive lesions, which was higher in the group of children without Down syndrome than in those with trisomy 21 (right-sided obstructions: 17% vs. 6%; left-sided obstructions: 11% vs. 2%).

CONCLUSIONS

Atrioventricular canal is the most common cardiac defect in patients with Down syndrome, usually occurring as an isolated defect with a low prevalence of obstructive lesions of the right or left ventricle. The early mortality for repair of atrioventricular canal has decreased since the 1980s as a result of improved methods of myocardial protection, better postoperative care, and better patient selection including the selective use of pulmonary artery banding. Early repair of atrioventricular canal should generally be performed between 6 and 12 months, and these results are comparable between patients with and without Down syndrome (2,10–12). Other lesions seen in patients with Down syndrome include an increased prevalence of inlet-type ventricular septal defect. Management and outcome of patients with Down syndrome with congenital heart defects are generally similar to those in patients with normal karyotype. Early intervention is indicated to prevent the development of irreversible pulmonary vascular disease, which may develop more rapidly in patients with Down syndrome.

REFERENCES

1. Clapp S, Perry BL, Farooki ZQ, et al. Down syndrome, complete atrioventricular canal, and pulmonary vascular obstructive disease. *J Thorac Cardiovasc Surg.* 1990;100:115–121.
2. Baciewicz FA, Basilius MD, Davis JT. Congenital heart disease in Down's patients: a decade of surgical experience. *J Thorac Cardiovasc Surg.* 1989;37:369–371.
3. De Biase L, Di Ciommo V, Ballerini L, Bevilacqua M, Marcelletti C, Marino B. Prevalence of left-sided obstructive lesions with atrioventricular canal without Down syndrome. *J Thorac Cardiovasc Surg.* 1986; 91:467–472.
4. Bharati S, Kirklin JW, McAllister HA, Lev M. The surgical anatomy of common atrioventricular orifice associated with tetralogy of Fallot, double-outlet ventricle and complete regular transposition. *Circulation.* 1980;61:1142–1149.
5. Berger TJ, Kirklin JW, Blakestone EH, et al. Primary repair of complete atrioventricular canal in patients less than two years old. *Am J Cardiol.* 1978;41:906–912.
6. Newfield EA, Sher M, Paul MH, Nikaidoh H. Pulmonary vascular disease in complete atrioventricular canal defects. *Am J Cardiol.* 1977;39: 721–726.

7. Berger TJ, Blakstone EH, Kirklin JW, et al. Survival and probability of cure without and with operation in complete atrioventricular canal. *Ann Thorac Surg.* 1979;27:104.

8. Bull C, Rigby M, Shinebourne EA. Should management of complete atrioventricular canal defect be influenced by coexistent Down's syndrome? *Lancet.* 1985;1:1147–1149.

9. Urban AE. Total correction of complete atrioventricular canal: surgical technique and analysis of long-term results. *Prog Pediatr Surg.* 1990; 25:118–122.

10. Midgley FM, Galioto FM, Shapiro SR, et al. Experience with repair of complete atrioventricular canal. *Ann Thorac Surg.* 1980;30(2):151–159.

11. Pozzi M, Remig J, Fimmers R, Urban AE. Atrioventricular septal defects. Analysis of short- and medium-term results. *J Thorac Cardiovasc Surg.* 1991;101:138–142.

12. Capouya E, Laks H, Perl JM. Technique of management of the left atrioventricular valve in the repair of atrioventricular orifice. *Cardiol Young.* 1991;1:356–366.

13. Sondheimar HM, Katrioventricularey RW, Blackman JW. Pulmonary artery banding as primary therapy for complete atrioventricular canal. *Pediatr Res.* 1978;78:28–33.

14. Epstein ML, Moller JH, Amplatz K, et al. Efficacy of pulmonary artery banding in infants with complete atrioventricular canal. *J Thorac Cardiovasc Surg.* 1979;78:28–31.

15. Silverman N, Levitsky S, Fisher E, et al. Efficacy of pulmonary artery banding in infants with complete atrioventricular canal. *Circulation.* 1983;68:ii148–53.

16. Chi TPL, Krovets LJ. The pulmonary vascular bed in children with Down syndrome. *J Pediatr.* 1975;86:533–538.

17. Studer M, Blackstone EH, Kirklin JW, et al. Determinants of early and late results of repair of atrioventricular septal (canal) defects. *J Thorac Cardiovasc Surg.* 1982;84:523–542.

18. McGrath LB, Gonzales-Lavin L. Actuarial survival, freedom from reoperation, and other events after repair of atrioventricular septal defects. *J Thorac Cardiovasc Surg.* 1987;94:582–590.

19. Bender HV, Hammon JV, Hubbard SG, et al. Repair of atrioventricular canal malformation in the first year of life. *J Thorac Cardiovasc Surg.* 1982;84:515–522.

20. William WH, Guyton RA, Michalik RE, et al. Individualized surgical management of complete atrioventricular canal. *J Thorac Cardiovasc Surg.* 1983;86:838–844.

21. Mair DD, McGoon DC. Surgical correction of atrioventricular canal during the first year of life. *Am J Cardiol.* 1977;40:66–69.

22. Bender HW, Hammon JW, Hubbard SG, et al. Repair of atrioventricular canal malformation in the first year of life. *J Thorac Cardiovasc Surg.* 1982;84:515–522.

23. Capouya ER, Laks HM, Drinkwater DC, Pearl JM, Milgalter E. Management of the left atrioventricular valve in the repair of complete atrioventricular septal defects. *J Thorac Cardiovasc Surg.* 1992;104: 196–203.

24. Carpentier A. Surgical anatomy and management of the mitral component of atrioventricular canal defects. In: Anderson AH, Shinebourne

EA, eds. *Pediatric Cardiology 1977*. Edinburgh: Churchill Livingstone; 1978:477–490.

25. Anderson RH, Zuberbuhler JR, Penkose PA, Neches WH. Of clefts, commissures, and things. *J Thorac Cardiovasc Surg*. 1985;90:605–610.
26. Starr A. Discussion of Bender et al. *J Thorac Cardiovasc Surg*. 1982; 84:515–522.
27. Castaneda AR, Mayer JE, Jonas RA. Repair of complete atrioventricular canal in infancy. *World J Surg*. 1985;9:590–597.
28. Bove EL, Sondhelmeer HM, Kavey RW, Byrum CJ, Blackman MS. Results with the two patch technique for repair of complete atrioventricular septal defects. *Ann Thorac Surg*. 1984;38:157–160.

—————— CHAPTER *15*——————

LONG-TERM FOLLOW-UP OF PERSONS WITH DOWN SYNDROME AND CONGENITAL HEART DISEASE

James B. Seward

In ORDER TO UNDERSTAND THE long-term impact of congenital heart disease on persons with Down syndrome, it is important to understand the natural history of congenital heart disease in patients without Down syndrome. It is estimated that 500,000 persons with congenital heart disease will reach adulthood in the United States by the year 2000. Thirty-eight percent of these adults will have had corrective surgery (1). It is also estimated that annually more than 8,500 young patients who have had cardiovascular surgery reach adulthood (2). Thus, an ever-increasing population with congenital heart disease is reaching adulthood, requiring cardiologists to become aware of the natural history of uncorrected as well as palliated and corrected congenital heart disease.

Patients with Down syndrome are no exception and studies are now reporting long survival of these individuals. In a large epidemiologic study of 2,328 random births, two chromosomal abnormalities were identified (3). Of 2,102 patients with cardiovascular abnormalities, 271 patients (12.9%) were found to have chromosomal abnormalities. Of the patients with Down syndrome affected with cardiovascular abnormalities, approximately 60% had an endocardial cushion defect. It was also noted that only 2.8% of patients with Down syndrome had an isolated cardiovascular defect. There is a high incidence of congenital cardiac disease in patients with Down syndrome, and the logical question is how this additional burden affects survival.

THE NATURAL HISTORY OF CONGENITAL
HEART DISEASE IN PATIENTS WITHOUT DOWN SYNDROME

First, it should be recognized that congenital heart disease begins during organogenesis (or during embryologic development). In an interesting study by Sharland, Lockhart, Chita, and Allan (4), the survival of 222 fetuses recognized as having congenital heart disease in the prenatal period was followed for 2 years (Figure 1). Approximately 25% of fetuses died in utero. An additional 45% died in the immediate neonatal period. By the end of infancy or early childhood, 75% of the 222 patients had died and only 47 were alive at follow-up. Only four of these patients had reached the age of 4 years. It becomes apparent that most natural history studies of congenital heart disease deal with children who have at least survived the fetal period; however, more often patients with congenital heart disease are studied from infancy and beyond. Thus, we may be missing 50%–75% of early mortality in patients with serious congenital heart disease.

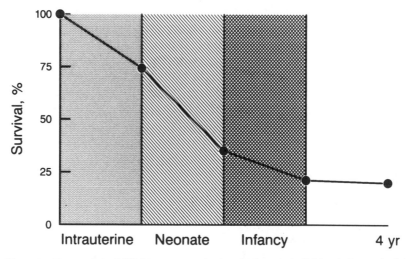

Figure 1. The survival of 222 fetuses recognized as having congenital heart disease in the prenatal period. Only four of these patients had reached the age of 4. Only 47 were alive at follow-up. (From Sharland GK, Lockhart SM, Chita SK, Allan LD. Factors influencing the outcome of congenital heart disease detected prenatally. *Arch Dis Child.* 1981;66(3):284–287. Reprinted by permission.)

If one looks at isolated studies regarding the survival of patients with Down syndrome having surgery for congenital heart disease, one can obtain a partial understanding of the natural history. In one study (5), 85 patients with Down syndrome and atrioventricular canal defect were investigated for survival. Of 49 patients with complete atrioventricular canal, 73% had Down syndrome. The overall survival for patients with Down syndrome and complete atrioventricular canal defect was 83%, whereas there was a statistical difference in the survival of patients with atrioventricular canal without Down syndrome (54%). This is contrasted with the partial atrioventricular canal (36 patients). The patients with Down syndrome represented only 14% of this group. There was a 95% overall survival with 100% of patients with Down syndrome surviving correction of partial atrioventricular canal. Thus, when considering the outcome survival of patients with Down syndrome it is necessary to distinguish less serious congenital cardiovascular anomalies from the more complex anomalies.

NATURAL HISTORY OF CONGENITAL HEART DISEASE

It is important to understand the long-term survival of patients without Down syndrome before embarking on a discussion of the long-term outcome of patients with Down syndrome associated with congenital heart disease. Two large series of patients give an overview of the natural history of congenital heart disease (6,7). Moller et al., from the University of Minnesota (7), assessed the long-term outcome of 1,000 consecutive patients undergoing surgical repair of congenital heart disease between 1952 and 1963. The follow-up was 26–37 years. Seventy-one percent of patients were alive at follow-up. The survival was directly related to 1) the complexity of the defect; 2) the year of the surgical repair, which reflected increasing surgical sophistication; and 3) late deaths in patients who had developed Eisenmenger syndrome. The latter group has some relevance to our understanding of the long-term survival of patients with Down syndrome. The authors further analyzed these 1,000 patients. Eighty-nine percent of survivors were asymptomatic and only 4% were on any drug therapy. Two conclusions can be extrapolated from this experience: 1) patients with Down syndrome with underlying complex disease and/or 2) pulmonary vascular obstructive disease will most adversely affect outcome.

The second large study is a multicenter natural history study that investigated a cadre of 2,408 patients with congenital heart disease from 1958 to 1988 (30 years of follow-up) (6). Three lesions were assessed including ventricular septal defect, pulmonary stenosis, and aortic stenosis. The natural history of ventricular septal defect in particular has relevance to the discussion of long-term outcome of patients with Down syndrome.

In patients with a ventricular septal defect, there was no significant variation in survival based on age of presentation. Younger patients initially had a slightly worse survival than those who presented later in life. This may reflect a more significant hemodynamic alteration in younger patients compared to those who remained asymptomatic or whose symptoms were undetected until later. Patients with ventricular septal defect had a slightly worse prognosis at 25 years than those with aortic stenosis and a significantly poorer prognosis than those with the more hemodynamically benign lesion of pulmonary stenosis. The survival of all patients with pulmonary stenosis did not show any significant difference from the expected survival at 25 years' follow-up. Patients with aortic stenosis, however, did have a significant variance from the expected survival as did patients with ventricular septal defect.

In order to address the issue of severity, each lesion was divided into subgroups based on hemodynamic severity. A 25-year follow-up of patients with pulmonary stenosis shows a significant difference in long-term survival based on severity of the gradient at presentation. This also holds true for aortic stenosis and ventricular septal defect. It should be noted that patients with a ventricular septal defect determined to be inoperable at initial presentation (i.e., Eisenmenger syndrome) had a 25-year survival of 40%.

In attempting to assess the natural history of patients with Down syndrome with congenital heart disease, these data must be taken into consideration. Patients with Down syndrome denied surgical intervention who develop Eisenmenger syndrome may be expected to have a relatively long survival even into the second or third decade of life. Two determinants that appear to affect survival most adversely are complexity or severity of the underlying lesion at presentation and long-term attrition attributable to pulmonary vascular disease. In the natural history study group, only those patients with Eisenmenger syndrome had a significant elevation of pulmonary artery pressure at follow-up.

The natural history study concluded the following: The possibility of a 25-year survival with isolated pulmonary stenosis was in excess of 96% and was not appreciably different from normal expected survival. Morbid events were rare and virtually all patients were in New York Heart Association Classification I. Four percent of the patients with a presenting gradient of less than 25 mm Hg progressed to operation. With each incremental increase in gradient, there was an increase in the probability of surgical intervention (gradient 25–49 mm Hg—21% to surgery, gradient 50–79 mm Hg—79% to surgery, gradient ≥80 mm Hg—97% to surgery). Surgical repair effectively lowered the gradient and reoperation was rare.

In patients with aortic stenosis, the probability of survival at 25 years was 85% of the total group and 92% if the presenting gradient was less than 50 mm Hg. Among the deaths, sudden death was the most common and was typically found in the group that was asymptomatic but with significant underlying disease. Serious ventricular arrhythmias were more often observed in patients with aortic stenosis than in the normal population, especially in patients with a high gradient either in the past or at presentation.

Small gradients invariably remained small and were best assessed by clinical examination and Doppler hemodynamics. Long-term surgical survivors had a mean gradient of 25 mm Hg by Doppler hemodynamics. At 25-year follow-up of the overall group, 32% were considered to be in excellent, 22% in good, 29% in fair, and 17% in poor health.

With regard to ventricular septal defect, patients with trivial, mild, and even moderate hemodynamic abnormalities were found to be in good functional status and their outlook for long-term survival was hardly different from that of the normal population. Patients with severe ventricular septal defect improved with surgical intervention; however, there was a higher rate of morbidity and mortality depending on the presenting severity. The most enlightening fact was that approximately 40% of patients presenting as inoperable (Eisenmenger syndrome) were alive at 25 years.

The natural history of congenital heart disease is further detailed in two additional studies, one dealing with isolated atrial septal defect (8) and the second dealing with postoperative Fontan procedure for complex congenital heart disease (9). For atrial septal defect, the postoperative life expectancy is completely normal and late complications are rare (8). Conversely, the natural history of complex congenital heart disease was much worse: 1-year survival was 77%; 5-year survival, 70%; and 10-year survival, 60%. Thirty percent of these patients required reoperation and 20% had demonstrable arrhythmia (9). These studies further illustrate the effect of the complexity of the underlying lesion or necessary operative repair on survival of congenital heart disease. In patients with Down syndrome, repair of partial atrioventricular canal has little appreciable effect on survival. Conversely, repair of complete atrioventricular canal is expected to have a significant effect on early and long-term survival. Children with complex congenital heart disease who are not operated on have an expected higher attrition over 3–5 decades.

NATURAL HISTORY OF DOWN SYNDROME AND CONGENITAL HEART DISEASE

There are only a few reports on the natural history of patients with Down syndrome surviving with congenital heart disease compared with the total population with Down syndrome. There is an interesting report from the California Department of Developmental Services that discusses the long-term survival of 13,567 patients with Down syndrome (10) (Figure 2). The investigators found that early in life there was a significant impact of congenital heart disease on the survival of patients with Down syndrome. However, after the first 4 or 5 years of life, the survival curves for patients with Down syndrome with and without congenital heart disease were nearly identical. The only group that separated out as a more significant predictor of survival was a group called "poor feeders," which comprised 11% of the total population with Down syndrome. These were patients who required supplemental feeding, had profound mental retardation, and

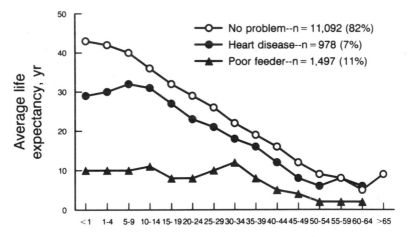

Figure 2. California Department of Developmental Services. Average life expectancy (in years) predicted from a cohort of 13,567 patients with Down syndrome. Findings indicate that the predictors of survival for people with Down syndrome were not different from the variables related to mortality among persons with mental retardation in general. A lack of mobility or feeding skills ("poor feeders") were better predictors of an early death than were medical problems associated with congenital heart disease. Life expectancy estimates of persons with Down syndrome who lacked mobility or eating skills were found to be poor compared to individuals who had Down syndrome but did not have these problems regardless of the presence of heart disease. (From Eyman P, Call TL, White JF. Life expectancy of persons with Down syndrome. *Am J Ment Retard.* 1991;95:603–612. Reprinted by permission.)

had significant musculoskeletal abnormalities. The poor feeders had a markedly reduced survival compared with patients with Down syndrome with or without cardiac problems. The investigators concluded that the survival of people with Down syndrome with or without congenital heart disease is not different from the mortality among people with mental retardation in general. Lack of mobility and feeding skills were better predictors of early death than the presence of congenital heart disease (10).

A study from the Cleveland Clinic (11) assessed the survival of patients with Down syndrome with cardiac disease having surgical or nonsurgical treatment over a 20-year follow-up. These investigators observed a high attrition (i.e., approximately 30% mortality) in the first 2–3 years of life. At the 20-year follow-up, the nonsurgical patients with Down syndrome and congenital heart disease had a significantly worse survival than those patients who had undergone surgical correction (Figure 3).

It is noted that the California Registry reported only 7% of its patients with Down syndrome as having congenital heart disease; however, reports gleaned primarily from tertiary medical centers suggest a much higher prevalence of congenital heart disease in patients with Down syndrome. Most series report approximately 40%–50% prevalence of congenital heart disease in infants with Down syndrome. The most common lesion is complete atrioventricular canal in approximately 33% of patients. These reports suggest that there is a lower survival of patients with congenital heart disease and that this

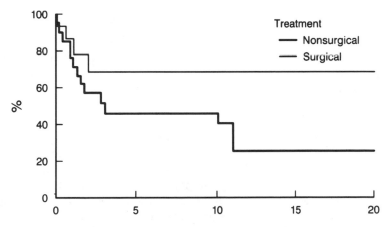

Figure 3. Twenty-year follow-up of patients with Down syndrome. Those patients undergoing surgical correction of congenital heart disease had a much better survival than those treated medically. (From Mathew P, et al. Long-term follow-up of children with Down syndrome with cardiac lesions. *Clin Pediatr.* 1990;29(10):569–574. Reprinted by permission.)

diminished survival can be improved with surgical repair (11,12). In one study, the 10-year survival of patients with Down syndrome with unoperated congenital heart disease was reported to be 53% whereas surgical survival was 83%. At 20 years, patients with unoperated congenital heart disease had 31% survival and with surgery 69% survival. A comparable assessment of patients with Down syndrome without congenital heart disease shows a 10-year survival of 77% and a 20-year survival of 71%. In a comparable general population, the expected 10-year survival is approximately 97% (11).

It is stated that life expectancy in patients with Down syndrome after the first 2–3 years of life is the same with or without congenital heart disease. With repair of congenital heart disease, survival can be expected well into the fifth, sixth, and seventh decades of life (12).

In a review of patients with Down syndrome with congenital heart disease undergoing echocardiographic examination at the Mayo Clinic, the only hemodynamic parameter that appeared to change with age was pulmonary artery pressure. Patients with Down syndrome with congenital heart disease surviving to age 20–40 years showed a significantly higher pulmonary artery pressure. This observation may be indirectly construed as a late manifestation of congenital heart disease. The 25-year survival of inoperable ventricular septal defect is over 40%. The increase of pulmonary artery pressure in the older patient reflects the natural evolution of the unoperated or delayed manifestation of congenital heart disease.

SUMMARY

A few assumptions regarding long-term survival of patients with Down syndrome can be made. First, congenital heart disease does have an impact on the natural history of surviving patients. Those with more complex lesions will have a worse survival than those with less complex cardiovascular abnormality. Patients with Down syndrome with partial atrioventricular canal have a survival quite similar to those without congenital heart disease, whereas patients with complete atrioventricular canal have a worse survival but are improved with surgical repair. The survival of unoperated congenital heart disease will depend on the severity of the underlying lesion and the hemodynamic consequence, primarily the development of pulmonary hypertension. However, even in patients who are inoperable or do not undergo surgery, survival can be quite long. Today it is not unusual to see patients with Down syndrome surviving into their 20s, 30s, or 40s with inoperable congenital heart disease. Patients with Down syndrome without significant residual congenital heart disease or serious manifestations of Down syndrome can be expected to have a much longer survival (i.e., well into the fifth, sixth, and seventh decades of life).

Patients with Down syndrome should be looked on as similar to the general population. Their survival is primarily related to the underlying presentation of Down syndrome and the magnitude of their mental and physical disabilities. Congenital heart disease is an added risk. There is a high attrition in the first 2 years of life secondary to the underlying syndrome, superimposed cardiovascular compromise, and corrective surgery. After this period the survival with or without congenital heart disease is similar. Only individuals with profound disabilities show an accelerated mortality. Death from underlying pulmonary vascular obstructive disease occurs slowly with many patients surviving well into adulthood. Patients with Down syndrome without congenital heart disease or a defect successfully repaired early in infancy can be expected to survive into the fourth and fifth decades of life. Surgery for congenital heart disease in patients with Down syndrome does modify the long-term survival. However, even patients without corrective surgery can be expected to have a significantly longer survival than had previously been predicted.

The data suggest that 1) patients with Down syndrome and heart disease are helped by cardiac surgery with stabilization and improvement of their functional class, 2) deterioration in functional class is seen in patients with Down syndrome with cardiac lesions who are managed surgically, and 3) mortality remains high in such patients treated nonsurgically due to the development of pulmonary vascular disease and congestive heart failure. Therefore, early diagnosis and surgical correction where appropriate is a key issue in the management of children with Down syndrome.

REFERENCES

1. Roberts NK, Cretin S. The changing face of congenital heart disease: a method of predicting the influence of cardiac surgery upon the prevalence and spectrum of congenital heart disease. *Med Care.* 1980;18: 930–939.
2. Morris CD, Menashe VD. 25-year mortality after surgical repair of congenital heart disease in childhood. *JAMA.* 1991;226:3447–3452.
3. Ferencz C, Neill CA, Boughman JA, Rubin JD, Brenner JI, Perry LW. Congenital cardiovascular malformations associated with chromosome abnormalities: an epidemiologic study. *J Pediatr.* 1989;114(1):79–86.
4. Sharland GK, Lockhart SM, Chita SK, Allan LD. Factors influencing the outcome of congenital heart disease detected prenatally. *Arch Dis Child.* 1981;66(3):284–287.

5. Vet TW, Ottenkamp J. Correction of atrioventricular septal defect. Results influenced by Down syndrome? *Am J Dis Child.* 1989;143(11): 1361–1365.

6. O'Fallon WM, Crowson CS, Rings LJ, et al. Second natural history study of congenital heart defects. *Circulation.* 1993;87(suppl I):I-4–15.

7. Moller JH, Anderson RC. Natural history of congenital heart disease: 1000 consecutive children with cardiac malformations with 26–37 year follow-up. *Am J Cardiol.* 1992;70:661–667.

8. Murphy J, Gersh B, McGoon M, et al. Long-term outcome after surgical repair of isolated atrial septal defect. *N Engl J Med.* 1990;323: 1645–1650.

9. Driscoll DJ, Offord KP, Feldt RH, Schaff HV, Puga FJ, Danielson GK. Five- to fifteen-year follow-up after Fontan operation. *Circulation.* 1992;85:469–496.

10. Eyman RK, Call TL, White JF. Life expectancy of persons with Down syndrome. *Am J Ment Retard.* 1991;95:603–612.

11. Mathew P, Moodie D, Sterba R, Murphy D, Rosenkranz E, Homa A. Long-term follow-up of children with Down syndrome with cardiac lesions. *Clin Pediatr.* 1990;29(10):569–574.

12. Baird PA, Sadovnick AD. Life expectancy in Down syndrome. *J Pediatr.* 1987;110:849–854.

—————————CHAPTER *16*—————————

CARDIAC FUNCTION OF PERSONS WITH DOWN SYNDROME WITHOUT CONGENITAL HEART DISEASE

James B. Seward

T HE INCIDENCE OF DOWN SYNDROME is 1 in 800–1,100 births. Of patients with Down syndrome, 40%–50% will have significant congenital heart disease, and only a small percentage of patients with Down syndrome with congenital heart disease will have an isolated defect (1). Rowe and Uchida (2) describe the cardiac malformations found in 70 patients with Down syndrome, the most common lesion being atrioventricular canal defect in 36% of the patients, with the majority of these being complete atrioventricular canal and a small percentage partial atrioventricular canal. Ventricular septal defect was found in 33%, ductus arteriosus in 10%, secundum atrial septal defect in 9%, isolated aberrant subclavian artery in 7%, tetralogy of Fallot in 1%, pulmonary stenosis in 1%, and other cardiac defects in 3% of patients. In general, the most common defects are atrioventricular canal defect, tetralogy of Fallot, and patent ductus arteriosus. Other complicating lesions, such as transposition of the great arteries, muscular ventricular septal defect, and complex atrioventricular canal, are noticeably absent.

It should also be reaffirmed that the clinical assessment of congenital heart disease in patients with Down syndrome should not rely on conventional clinical examination, chest X-ray, and electrocardiogram. The echocardiogram is the best screening examination for congenital heart disease in patients with Down syndrome (3).

SURVIVAL OF PATIENTS WITH DOWN SYNDROME

The literature is interesting with regard to survival of patients with Down syndrome. Articles published in the 1930s and 1950s describe a survival of less than 20 years (5–6). By the mid-1980s, survival was described as greater than 40 years in 40%–50% of patients (7). Now in the late 1980s and early 1990s, survival is considered to be quite long with more than 50% of persons with Down syndrome living more than 50 years (8,9). If you look specifically at patients with Down syndrome with congenital heart disease (10), survival is adversely affected by the severity of the underlying congenital heart disease: 50% of patients with congenital heart disease will survive beyond the age of 30 years, compared with 79% of those without congenital heart disease surviving beyond 30 years. Based on the long-term follow-up of 13,567 patients with Down syndrome without cardiac problems, many survived into the fifth, sixth, and seventh decades of life (11). Congenital heart disease identified early in life had a significant impact on survival; however, when congenital heart disease was diagnosed after the age of 5 years, patients with Down syndrome with congenital heart disease had a subsequent survival similar to those without congenital heart disease. The primary impact on survival was severe retardation, difficulty maintaining nutrition, and other associations such as musculoskeletal disability. A study from the California Department of Developmental Services (11) states that lack of mobility or feeding skills was a better predictor of survival than associated congenital heart disease. Patients with Down syndrome with good mobility and feeding skills have a survival no different from that of individuals with mental retardation of other etiology.

SURVIVAL WITHOUT SURGERY
FOR CONGENITAL HEART DISEASE

In patients with Down syndrome and significant congenital heart disease who do not undergo surgery, the primary disability is that of the development of pulmonary vascular obstructive disease. It is stated that fixed obstructive pulmonary disease is present in approximately

12% of patients with Down syndrome younger than 1 year of age, whereas it was found in 0% of patients without Down syndrome (12). From these data it is apparent that pulmonary vascular disease progresses at an accelerated rate in patients with Down syndrome (13). Medical concerns observed in late life are primarily related to pneumonia (31%–76% of patients), congestive heart failure (31%–56% of patients), and pulmonary vascular disease (25% of patients with Down syndrome in less than a year). On the basis of these observations, surgical intervention is recommended early in order to avert complications of pulmonary vascular disease. However, one should remember that the natural history study of inoperable ventricular septal defect (Eisenmenger syndrome) indicated that approximately 40% of these patients will have a survival of 25 years (14). Thus, even the unoperated patient with Down syndrome with pulmonary vascular obstructive disease will have a fairly long survival (see also Chapter 15).

The highest mortality in patients with Down syndrome with congenital heart disease is in the first 3 months of life with an operative mortality nominally reported as 10%–20% (15). A delay in surgery results in a rapid rise in the prevalence of pulmonary vascular obstructive disease. By 2 years of age, 88% of patients with Down syndrome with underlying significant congenital heart disease have inoperable pulmonary vascular disease. Early mortality with congenital heart disease in patients with Down syndrome is high (16). The reported mortality of patients with Down syndrome undergoing surgical correction of congenital heart disease was 16.4% at 30 days and 27.3% at 33 months (17). However, after this initial attrition, long-term survival of operated patients with Down syndrome is quite satisfactory. In a review of 126 patients from the Mayo Clinic, the age of presentation for anatomic and hemodynamic assessment of patients with Down syndrome was predominantly less than 1 year. After the first year the frequency of necessary cardiovascular surgery throughout life is low. This is thought to reflect a high prevalence of early mortality and early definitive surgery in patients with Down syndrome.

By separating patients with Down syndrome undergoing surgery into groups of less than 11 years of age and one more than 11 years of age, it can be seen that surgery in the younger patient group reduced the necessity for subsequent surgery. When the indications for surgery are further scrutinized, it can be seen that no patient 11 years and older had correction of a major cardiovascular anomaly. Two patients in the Mayo Clinic series who were older than 11 years had partial atrioventricular canal repaired, one patient had cardiac surgery for simple atrial septal defect, and four others had minor cardiovascular surgery. All significant congenital heart diseases were operated on early in childhood with an associated early attrition. Early mortality was primarily related to the severity of the underlying cardiovascular anomaly (i.e., complete atrioventricular canal, ventricular septal defect, tetralogy of Fallot). At approximately 8 years' follow-up, the survival of the surgical group is increased over the survival of the nonsurgical group (9). Patients with congenital heart disease who did not undergo cardiac surgery have a reduced early survival and those who have mild congenital cardiac abnormalities do well.

The most significant attrition due to congenital heart disease occurs in the first 2–5 years of life. After this early attrition, long-term survival is similar to that of the general population of patients with Down syndrome without congenital heart disease (11). The survival curve of patients with Down syndrome with congenital heart disease after approximately 1 year begins to look like that of the patient without congenital heart disease (18).

VENTRICULAR FUNCTION/PULMONARY PRESSURE

If one examines the left ventricular function as assessed by echocardiography in young and adult patients with Down syndrome, one finds that the left ventricular size and systolic function are not appreciably different between young and adult. In 126 patients followed at the Mayo Clinic, we found no significant difference in ventricular dimensions and ejection fraction in the first 5 decades of life. The only significant observation was in the unoperated patient, which reflects the increased prevalence of pulmonary vascular obstructive disease in the unoperated patient with Down syndrome who developed an elevation of pulmonary artery pressure. This reflects the increased prevalence of pulmonary vascular obstructive disease in the unoperated patient. The most significant difference is between the surgical and nonsurgical groups relative to pulmonary artery pressure. The highest pulmonary artery pressures were observed in patients age 21–40. There appears to be an attrition of this group of patients, since by the fifth decade of life we no longer see a significant difference between pulmonary artery pressure in the nonsurgical and surgical groups. When we studied survival by age, we found that the majority of deaths in the Mayo Clinic group occurred in the first year of life. Ninety-one percent of all deaths occurred in the surgical group. Only 9% of those medically treated died at less than 1 year of age. However, subsequent deaths occurred only in the medically treated group and began to occur after the age of 20 years, which reflects the attrition primarily due to pulmonary vascular obstructive disease.

The impact of congenital heart disease on survival of patients with Down syndrome is significant and appears to most adversely affect survival in patients less than 1 year of age and in the older unoperated group. In the third and fourth decades of life, death occurred secondary to progressive hemodynamic insult of pulmonary vascular obstructive disease. Those patients without congenital heart disease have a long survival and their outcome is primarily related to the secondary manifestations of Down syndrome (i.e., mental retardation and musculoskeletal disability) (10). According to available data, cardiac function is not appreciably different from that of the unaffected population. There is no increase in cardiac dimension or decrease in systolic ventricular function. The only observed longitudinal abnormality was increasing pulmonary vascular obstructive disease in a certain subset of unoperated patients with Down syndrome. Patients with Down syndrome considered inoperable had a reasonably long survival (see also Chapters 12 and 13).

SUMMARY

The patients with Down syndrome without congenital heart disease can be expected to have a reasonably long survival (11). That survival is directly related to the degree of underlying secondary manifestation of Down syndrome (i.e., magnitude of mental retardation, feeding problems, and musculoskeletal disability). Those patients with associated congenital heart disease break down into three groups: 1) those with early presentation requiring surgery; 2) those allocated to no surgery or considered inoperable; and 3) those with minor cardiovascular abnormalities, such as isolated primum atrial septal defect. The first-year mortality is very high and directly related to the severity of the underlying cardiovascular abnormality, the attendant surgical risk, and the postoperative management. Newer surgical techniques can reduce this risk considerably but still place patients with Down syndrome at a greater risk than the general population with the same underlying congenital malformation. After the first or second year of life, the survival curve for patients with operated congenital heart disease is nearly identical to that for patients with Down syndrome without congenital heart disease. The unoperated group develops progressive pulmonary vascular obstructive disease; however, it is predicted that a high percentage of these patients will live 10–20 years or more. The only identifiable long-term hemodynamic or functional cardiovascular abnormality is the development of pulmonary artery hypertension. The ethical and social problems of management of Down syndrome can only be addressed on a patient-by-patient basis. Early surgical intervention does result in a lowered long-term risk of pulmonary vascular obstructive disease. Survival after the first year or two of life is expectedly long and related primarily to the Down syndrome and development of pulmonary vascular obstructive disease.

REFERENCES

1. Ferencz C, Neill CA, Boughman JA, Rubin JD, Brenner JI, Perry LW. Congenital cardiovascular malformations associated with chromosome abnormalities: an epidemiologic study. *J Pediatr.* 1989;114:79–86.
2. Rowe RD, Uchida IA. Cardiac malformations in mongolism: a prospective study of 184 mongoloid children. *Am J Med.* 1961;31:726–735.
3. Tubman TRJ, Shields MD, Craig BG, Mulholland HC, Nevin NC. Congenital heart disease in Down's syndrome: two-years' prospective early screening study. *Br Heart J.* 1991;302:1425–1427.
4. Penrose LS. The incidence of mongolism in the general population. *J Ment Sci.* 1949;95:685–688.
5. Dayton N, Doering CR, Hilferty MM, Maher HC, Dolan HH. Mortality and expectation of life in mental deficiency in Massachusetts: analysis of the fourteen-year period, 1917–1930. *N Engl J Med.* 1932;206: 555–570.
6. Malzberg B. Life tables for patients with mental disease. *Mental Hyg.* 1932;16:464–480.
7. Thase ME. Longevity and mortality in Down's syndrome. *J Ment Defic Res.* 1982;26:177–192.
8. Dupont A, Vaeth M, Videback P. Mortality and life expectancy of Down's syndrome in Denmark. *J Ment Defic Res.* 1986;30:111–120.
9. Eyman RK, Grossman HJ, Tarjan G, Miller C. *Life expectancy and mental retardation.* Monograph No. 7. Washington, DC: American Association on Mental Deficiency; 1987.
10. Baird PA, Sadovnick AD. Life expectancy in Down syndrome. *J Pediatr.* 1987;110:849–854.
11. Eyman RK, Call TL, White JF. Life expectancy of persons with Down syndrome. *Am J Ment Retard.* 1991;95(6):603–612.
12. Mathew P, Moodie D, Sterba R, Murphy D, Rosenkranz E, Homa A. Long term follow-up of children with Down syndrome with cardiac lesions. *Clin Pediatr.* 1990;29:569–574.
13. Baird PA, Sadovnick AD. Causes of death to age 30 in Down syndrome. *Am J Hum Genet.* 1988;43:239–248.
14. O'Fallon WM, Crowson CS, Rings LJ, et al. Second natural history study of congenital heart defects. *Circulation.* 1992;87(suppl I):14–15.
15. Thieren M, Stijns-Cailteux M, Tremoroux-Wattiez M, et al. Congenital heart disease and obstructive pulmonary vascular diseases in Down's syndrome. Apropos of 142 children with trisomy 21. *Arch Mal Coeur Vaiss.* 1988;81(5):655–661.
16. Baciewicz FA Jr, Melvin WS, Basilius D, Davis JT. Congenital heart disease in Down's syndrome patients: a decade of surgical experience. *Thorac Cardiovasc Surg.* 1989;37(6):369–371.

17. Mathew P, Moodie D, Sterba R, Murphy D, Rosenkranz E, Homa A. Long-term follow-up of children with Down syndrome with cardiac lesions. *Clin Pediatr.* 1990;29:569–574.
18. Mastroiacovo P, Bertollini R, Corchia C. Survival of children with Down syndrome in Italy. *Am J Med Genet.* 1992;42(2):208–212.

MITRAL VALVE PROLAPSE AND AORTIC REGURGITATION IN ADULTS WITH DOWN SYNDROME

Siegfried M. Pueschel

T HE CHAPTERS IN THIS BOOK demonstrate that congenital heart disease in children with Down syndrome has been investigated extensively during past decades. Approximately a century ago, Garrod brought to the attention of the scientific community the increased prevalence of congenital heart disease in children with Down syndrome (1). Since then numerous publications have characterized various aspects of cardiac concerns in these children. As this volume documents, cardiologists have primarily focused on congenital heart disease and cardiac functions in children with Down syndrome, and only a few studies have been concerned with cardiac manifestations in adults with this chromosome abnormality.

There are several reasons for the paucity of information available in the medical literature pertaining to cardiologic defects in adults with Down syndrome. Prior to 1970, few individuals with Down syndrome survived early childhood. This was particularly true for those who resided in institutions. Only 25 years ago the life expectancy of persons with Down syndrome was about one fourth of that observed in the 1990s (2,3). Moreover, previously many children with severe congenital heart disease succumbed during the first few years of life, and those who survived were rarely monitored appropriately by medical personnel during adolescence and adulthood. Only since the

1970s has cardiac surgery for children with Down syndrome become widely available; and subsequently, more sophisticated diagnostic techniques (as well as compassionate and rational medical care) have been introduced. Thus, not enough time has passed for well-controlled longitudinal follow-up studies to be performed with regard to adults with Down syndrome. Furthermore, because the adults with Down syndrome and without congenital heart disease usually did not have significant cardiac problems, there was no apparent need for cardiac investigations regarding these persons. Only in recent years have a few investigators paid attention to cardiac functions in adults with Down syndrome.

MITRAL VALVE PROLAPSE AND AORTIC INSUFFICIENCY IN PERSONS WITH DOWN SYNDROME

Goldhaber and coworkers examined the cardiac status of 131 adults with Down syndrome who were residing in a large state institution for persons with mental retardation (4). For the purposes of this study, clinical heart disease was defined as an abnormally wide or fixed split-second sound, a systolic click, a Grade III/VI systolic precordial murmur, or any diastolic precordial murmur. Using these criteria, 38 (29%) of 131 patients with Down syndrome were found to have clinical heart disease. In order to confirm and evaluate the auscultatory findings, echocardiographic examinations were done on 37 patients. Eight patients with Down syndrome were found to have aortic regurgitation. All eight patients had high-frequency diastolic vibration of the anterior mitral valve as shown on echocardiography. The only manifestation of clinical heart disease in five of the eight patients was isolated aortic regurgitation. In addition to the observed aortic regurgitation, the other three individuals had ventricular septal defect, healed aortic and mitral valve endocarditis, and mitral valve prolapse, respectively. Of the 38 patients with clinical heart disease, eighteen were found by both physical examination and echocardiography, to have mitral valve prolapse. In 11 patients, mitral valve prolapse occurred as an isolated cardiac abnormality, and in two patients there was a systolic click without a systolic murmur. Three patients had echocardiographic evidence of tricuspid valve prolapse, and 11 patients with clinical heart disease had atrial or ventricular septal defects (4).

A subsequent case control study by Goldhaber and coinvestigators was designed to determine whether mitral valve prolapse and aortic regurgitation are observed at higher frequencies in persons with Down syndrome than in individuals with mental retardation due to other etiologies (5). The cohort of 131 persons with Down syndrome who were identified in the authors' first publication served as the study group; individuals from the same institution in whom mental retardation was the result of low birthweight or perinatal asphyxia constituted the control group. Cardiac examinations were performed prospectively in all 92 control patients using the same clinical criteria for the presence of clinical heart disease as employed in Goldhaber's previous study (4). If significant heart disease was noted, two-dimensional and M-mode echocardiography were carried out. Goldhaber and his group found mitral valve prolapse in 14% of persons with Down syndrome but in only 4% of the control group members ($p = 0.02$). Aortic regurgitation was observed in 6% of the individuals with Down syndrome and in 2% of the control group patients ($p = 0.16$). Thus, the relative risk of mitral valve prolapse in persons with Down syndrome was 3.5 and that of aortic regurgitation was 2.9, indicating that these two valvular abnormalities are specifically associated with Down syndrome in adulthood (5).

In another study, Goldhaber and coworkers examined 35 asymptomatic adults with Down syndrome who did not reside in institutions (6). During these evaluations, brief cardiac histories, readings of systemic arterial pressure, and heart rates were obtained along with cardiac auscultation and Doppler echocardiography. Mitral valve prolapse was considered to be present when the systolic mitral valve leaflet motion continued beyond the plane of the mitral valve anulus into the left atrium from all three of the following views: the parasternal long axis and apical two- and four-chamber views. Aortic regurgitation was identified by Doppler echocardiography as high-velocity retrograde blood flow in the left ventricular outflow tract throughout diastole and by M-mode echocardiography as high-frequency diastolic vibration of the mitral valve. Goldhaber found that 10 of the 35 subjects with Down syndrome had normal cardiac auscultation and normal two-dimensional echocardiograms (6). Twenty individuals (57%) had mitral valve prolapse. In 18 of the 20 subjects, mitral valve prolapse was associated with a midsystolic click or midsystolic murmur. Echocardiograms demonstrated that the mitral valve prolapse was holosystolic. Five of the 20 subjects with mitral valve prolapse also had associated tricuspid valve prolapse. No mitral valve regurgitation was observed. The aortic valves of most subjects were within normal limits, and only four of the 35 patients had Doppler echocardiographic evidence of aortic regurgitation. Thus, among 35 noninstitutionalized adults with Down syndrome, 57% had mitral valve prolapse and 11% had aortic regurgitation (6).

Another group of investigators examined 83 noninstitutionalized, randomly selected patients with Down syndrome who were between the ages of 9 and 55 years (7). The authors reported that 41 of the

83 patients had echocardiographic findings indicative of mitral valve prolapse and that 15 of these patients lacked associated auscultatory findings.

Pueschel and Werner designed a study to determine the prevalence of mitral valve prolapse and aortic insufficiency in 36 young persons with Down syndrome between the ages of 18 and 32 years who had resided in home settings (8). Routine cardiac examinations revealed that all 36 patients had regular sinus rhythms. The first heart sound was normal in all patients; however, the second heart sound was accentuated in 12 of the 36 patients and widely split in six of them. Cardiac murmurs were heard in 11 patients: a Grade I/VI murmur was heard in six, a Grade II/VI murmur in four, and a Grade III/VI murmur was heard in one. Of the 36 individuals with Down syndrome enrolled in this study, 16 had normal echocardiograms and 20 had abnormal echocardiographic findings. Thirteen patients had mitral valve prolapse; in addition, three had both mitral valve prolapse and aortic insufficiency, two had only aortic insufficiency, and two had other mitral valve disorders. (One had thickening of the anterior leaflet of the mitral valve without prolapse, and the other had a partial cleft mitral valve). In 14 of the 16 patients with mitral valve prolapse, a midsystolic click was heard on auscultation. In nine individuals, the mitral valve prolapse was in midsystole; in the remaining seven patients holosystolic mitral valve prolapse was noted. Mitral insufficiency was noted in four of the patients with mitral valve prolapse (8).

Thus, the studies reported to date reveal that mitral valve prolapse occurs in 44%–57% of adults with Down syndrome, and aortic regurgitation in 11%–14% of adults with Down syndrome. Why do persons with Down syndrome have a higher frequency of mitral valve prolapse and aortic regurgitation? According to Washington and Allen, the precise cause of mitral valve prolapse is not known (9). The authors mention several possible causes of mitral valve prolapse, incuding rheumatic heart disease, connective tissue disorders, cardiomyopathies, and congenital heart disease. They then suggest that the primary lesion associated with mitral valve prolapse and aortic regurgitation appears to be a degeneration of the leaflets and chordae. A lengthening of the chordae then results, precipitating the prolapse of the mitral valve apparatus (9).

THE ETIOLOGY OF MITRAL VALVE PROLAPSE IN PERSONS WITH DOWN SYNDROME

Because mitral valve prolapse has been associated with syndromes characterized by weakness or laxity of connective tissue (e.g., Marfan syndrome, Ehlers-Danlos syndrome), it is possible that the increased prevalence of mitral valve prolapse and aortic insufficiency in adults with Down syndrome is due to a connective tissue disorder. It is widely known that general ligamentous laxity is prevalent in individuals with Down syndrome. Furthermore, higher frequencies of hip dislocation, patellar subluxation, and atlantoaxial instability are observed in individuals with Down syndrome; these higher frequencies are assumed to be the results of the increased ligamentous laxity (10). The same collagen tissues that surround the joints of the hip, knees, and cervical spine may also be present in the valvular structures of the heart.

Previous investigations indicate that children with Down syndrome may have an intrinsic defect of the connective tissue that results in increased ligamentous laxity (11). More recent studies have found decreased collagen fiber density of infiltrative connective tissues in persons with Down syndrome (12). Of importance is also the report by Duff, Williamson, and Richards, who demonstrated the expression of genes that had been mapped to the Down syndrome region of chromosome 21 and that encode two chains of the extracellular matrix molecule collagen type-IV in human fetal heart tissue using Northern blot analysis (13).

CLINICAL IMPLICATIONS

According to Goldhaber et al., the increased frequency of mitral valve prolapse and aortic regurgitation in persons with Down syndrome may have important clinical implications (6). In order to prevent endocarditis, it is generally recommended that adults with Down syndrome who have mitral valve prolapse and aortic regurgitation be provided with antibiotic prophylaxis before dental procedures and before any form of surgical intervention. Goldhaber et al. stated that antibiotic prophylaxis is particularly relevant to individuals with Down syndrome because they are very susceptible to periodontal disease (6). According to Barnett, Friedman, and Kastner, mitral valve prolapse may predispose patients to bacterial endocarditis after bacteremia-producing dental procedures. The authors state that if only auscultatory findings are used, a large number of persons with Down syndrome who are at risk for endocarditis may not be identified during routine physical examination (7).

MITRAL VALVE PROLAPSE IN RELATION TO SPORT ACTIVITIES AND EXERCISES

Because many persons with Down syndrome engage in recreational and competitive sport activities, the possibility of a connection between mitral valve prolapse and significant morbidity in individuals with Down syndrome should be explored. Although no information is available concerning the long-term effect of mitral valve prolapse in persons with Down syndrome who participate in sport activities such as the Special Olympics, there are a few reports in the medical literature that discuss the results of exercises in persons with mitral valve prolapse who do not have Down syndrome. Gallo and coinvestigators evaluated the autonomic nervous system of the heart in male patients with mitral valve prolapse (14). These investigators found that sinus arrhythmia was more often observed in patients with mitral valve prolapse than the members of a control group who did not have mitral valve prolapse. However, during the dynamic exercise test, no significant difference was noted between the study and control groups. The investigators concluded that the parasympathetic abnormalities in their patients with mitral valve prolapse, if present, are of questionable physiologic significance and generally would not affect the sympathetic and parasympathetic control of the heart rate during dynamic exercise (14).

In another study, Drory, Fisman, Pines, and Kellerman assessed the exercise response in 198 young women with echocardiographically documented mitral valve prolapse (15). Compared with 105 age- and sex-matched persons who did not have mitral valve prolapse, the individuals with mitral valve prolapse had a significantly higher mean heart rate, systolic blood pressure, pulse pressure, and rate pressure at rest and during exercise. The latter group also had a significantly lower mean maximal physical working capacity and a significantly higher prevalence of both arrhythmias and nonspecific ST and T wave changes as well as a significantly lower mean corrected QT interval. None of these findings, however, were associated with physical symptoms or with specific auscultatory or echocardiographic findings. The investigations of Drory et al. suggest that there is an autonomic nervous system imbalance in some young women with mitral valve prolapse irrespective of whether physical symptoms are present (15).

According to Washington and Allen, isolated mitral valve prolapse appears to be a relatively benign disorder (9). There may be complications, however, which include endocarditis, ventricular or atrial dysrhythmias, cerebral vascular accidents, congestive heart failure, severe chest pain, and sudden death. Washington and Allen indicate that although these complications are very rare, individuals with mitral valve prolapse should be monitored yearly (9).

Also, Jeresaty mentioned that the prognosis of mitral valve prolapse is generally favorable with regard to athletic activities (16). Although the author emphasized that infrequent complications may occur (e.g., transient ischemic attacks, progression of mitral regurgitation with or without ruptured chordae tendineae, infective endocarditis, sudden death), these symptoms or complications are not usually related to physical activity. The author believed that although a permissive attitude toward participation of patients with mitral valve prolapse in competitive sport activities is probably warranted, it is prudent to disqualify athletes with mitral valve prolapse when they have histories of syncope, acute chest pain, complex ventricular arrhythmias, mitral regurgitation, prolonged QT intervals, or a family history of sudden death (16).

Although many authors do not consider mitral valve prolapse findings in the majority of patients to be a serious disorder, Düren, Becker, and Dunning reported that 100 of 300 patients with mitral valve prolapse developed complications, including sudden death (three patients), ventricular tachycardia (56 patients), infective endocarditis (eight patients), and cerebral vascular accidents (11 patients) (17). Based on their data, the investigators suggest that the outlook for patients with mitral valve prolapse may not be as benign as described by other authors (17).

In 1992, Pitetti and coworkers compared the cardiovascular capacities of individuals with Down syndrome with those of persons with mental retardation due to other etiologies (18). These investigators found that individuals without Down syndrome had significantly higher mean peak oxygen consumption, minute ventilation measures, and heart rates than persons with Down syndrome. When walking at a speed of 3 miles per hour, subjects with Down syndrome had a significantly increased mean cardiac output, heart rate, and left ventricular work index, as well as a lower peripheral vascular resistance than those without Down syndrome (18). In contrast, when conducting cardiovascular fitness testing, Fernhall, Tymeson, Miller, and Burkett did not observe any cardiovascular abnormalities during exhaustive work in subjects with Down syndrome (19). These authors concluded that persons with Down syndrome can safely engage in rigorous exercise programs provided they are prescreened for exercise contraindications and are carefully supervised. The investigators of the latter two studies did not report whether or not some of the persons with Down syndrome had mitral valve prolapse (18,19).

It is generally assumed that the majority of individuals with Down syndrome who have been diagnosed with mitral valve prolapse will be asymptomatic and will be able to compete in sport activities without harmful effects. However, individuals who display arrhythmias, syncope, mitral insufficiency, chest pain, specific electrocardiographic abnormalities, or other mitral valve defects should refrain from participation in sport activities. Further studies are needed in order to evaluate the long-term effect of mitral valve prolapse and/or aortic insufficiency in persons with Down syndrome in relation to sport activities.

REFERENCES

1. Garrod AE. On the association of cardiac malformation with other congenital defects. *St. Bart Hosp Rep.* 1894;30:53–61.
2. Fabia J, Drolette M. Life tables up to age 10 for mongols with and without congenital heart defect. *J Ment Defic Res.* 1970;14:235–242.
3. Sadovnick AD, Baird PA. Life expectancy. In: Pueschel SM, Pueschel JK, eds. *Biomedical Concerns in Persons with Down Syndrome.* Baltimore: Paul H. Brookes Publishing Co.; 1992:47–57.
4. Goldhaber SZ, Rubin IL, Brown WD, Robertson N, Stubblefield F, Sloss LJ. Valvular heart disease (aortic regurgitation and mitral valve prolapse) among institutionalized adults with Down's syndrome. *Am J Cardiol.* 1986;57:278–281.
5. Goldhaber SZ, Brown WD, Robertson N, Rubin IL, St. John Sutton NG. Aortic regurgitation and mitral valve prolapse with Down's syndrome: a case-controlled study. *J Ment Defic Res.* 1988;32:333–336.
6. Goldhaber SZ, Brown WD, St. John Sutton NG. High frequency of mitral valve prolapse and aortic regurgitation among asymptomatic adults with Downs syndrome. *JAMA.* 1987;258:1793–1795.
7. Barnett ML, Friedman D, Kastner T. The prevalence of mitral valve prolapse in patients with Down's syndrome: implications for dental management. *Oral Surg Oral Med Oral Pathol.* 1988;66:445–447.
8. Pueschel SM, Werner JC. Mitral valve prolapse in persons with Down syndrome. *Res Dev Disabil.* (in press).
9. Washington RL, Allen S. How to manage mitral valve prolapse in children. *Your Patient and Fitness.* 1990;4:4–8.
10. Pueschel SM, Solga PM. Musculoskeletal disorders. In: Pueschel SM, Pueschel JK, eds. *Biomedical Concerns in Persons with Down Syndrome.* Baltimore: Paul H. Brookes Publishing Co.; 1992:147–157.
11. Pueschel SM, Scola FH, Perry CD, Pezzullo JC. Atlanto-axial instability in children with Down's syndrome. *J Ped Radiol.* 1981;10:129–132.
12. Reuland-Bosma W, Liem RS, Yansen HW, Van Dijk LJ, Van der Weele LT. Cellular aspects of and effect on the gingiva in children with Down's syndrome during experimental gingivitis. *J Clin Periodontol.* 1988;15:303–311.
13. Duff K, Williamson R, Richards JS. Expression of genes encoding two chains of the collagen type VI molecule. *Inter J Cardiol.* 1990;27:128–129.
14. Gallo DL, Morelo-Filho J, Maciel BC, Marine-Neto JA, Martins LE, Lima-Filho EC, Terra-Filho J, Almeida-Filho OC, Pintya AO, Manco JC. Evaluation of the autonomic nervous system of the heart in male patients with mitral valve prolapse syndrome using respiratory sinus arrhythmia and dynamic exercise. *Cardiol.* 1989;76:433–441.
15. Drory Y, Fisman EZ, Pines A, Kellerman JJ. Exercise response in young women with mitral valve prolapse. *Chest.* 1989;96:1076–1080.

16. Jeresaty RM. Mitral valve prolapse: definition and implication in athletes. *J Am Coll Cardiol.* 1986;7:231–236.
17. Düren DR, Becker AE, Dunning AJ. Long term follow up of idiopathic mitral valve prolapse in 300 patients: a prospective study. *J Am Coll Cardiol.* 1988;11:42–47.
18. Pitetti KH, Climstein M, Campbell KD, Barrett PJ, Jackson JA. The cardiovascular capacities of adults with Down syndrome: a comparative study. *Med Sci Sports and Exerc.* 1992;24:13–19.
19. Fernhall B, Tymeson GT, Miller L, Burkett LN. Cardiovascular fitness testing and fitness levels of adolescents and adults with mental retardation including Down syndrome. *Educ Train Ment Retard.* 1989; 133–138.

INDEX

Page numbers in *italic* denote figures; those followed by *t* denote tables.